Domestic Violence

One in four women will experience violence in the home at least once in their lives and many will be subjected to long-term violence. Health care practitioners are very often the first people to identify a problem related to domestic violence, but little has been published to support them in understanding what to do next. This handbook not only provides a clear introduction to the theoretical debates surrounding the topic but also offers practical advice on possible interventions. Focusing on improving the care of clients it covers:

- the causes and consequences of domestic violence
- personal and professional issues for the practitioner
- domestic violence and the law
- the process of effective intervention
- interventions in specific health care settings
- interventions where children are involved
- multi-agency approaches
- education and training.

Taking an evidence-based approach to practical problems, *Domestic Violence – A Handbook for Health Professionals* will be a welcome new resource for nurses, doctors and other health practitioners who deal with the consequences of domestic violence in their daily work. It will also be of interest to police, legal services, and those working in social services and voluntary organizations, such as Citizens' Advice Bureaux and victim support groups.

Lyn Shipway, Principal Lecturer in the School of Health Care Practice, has 18 years experience teaching health care students. Previously a night sister with expertise in Accident and Emergency, Orthopaedic, and Paediatric nursing, she has long had an interest in working with students to explore the psychological and social needs of various client groups as well as their biological health deficits.

40667

UHL NHS Trust - libraries

Domestic Violence

GLENFIELD
MEDICAL LIBRARY

A handbook for health professionals

Lyn Shipway

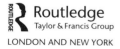

Routledge
Taylor & Francis Group

LONDON AND NEW YORK

First published 2004
by Routledge
11 New Fetter Lane, London EC4P 4EE

Simultaneously published in the USA and Canada
by Routledge
29 West 35th Street, New York, NY 10001

Routledge is an imprint of the Taylor & Francis Group

© 2004 Lyn Shipway

Typeset in Goudy and Gill by BC Typesetting Ltd, Bristol
Printed and bound in Great Britain by
TJ International Ltd, Padstow, Cornwall

All rights reserved. The purchase of this copyright material confers the right on
the purchasing institution to photocopy pages 195–198; 202–204; and 213–214
only. No other part of this book may be reprinted or reproduced or utilized in
any form or by any electronic, mechanical, or other means, now known or
hereafter invented, including photocopying and recording, or in any information
storage or retrieval system, without permission in writing from the publishers.

Every effort has been made to ensure that the advice and information in this
book is true and accurate at the time of going to press. However, neither the
publisher nor the authors can accept any legal responsibility or liability for any
errors or omissions that may be made. In the case of drug administration, any
medical procedure or the use of technical equipment mentioned within this
book, you are strongly advised to consult the manufacturer's guidelines.

British Library Cataloguing in Publication Data
A catalogue record for this book is available from the British Library

Library of Congress Cataloging in Publication Data
A catalog record for this book has been requested

ISBN 0–415–28206–3 (hbk)
ISBN 0–415–28220–9 (pbk)

For my son Andrew, and my daughter Emma-Lucy, who are the 'wind beneath my wings'

This book is dedicated to women and children everywhere who daily survive in a home where fear is the norm but where hope remains eternal. It is also dedicated to those individuals and groups who work relentlessly to impact on and improve the lives of those who are being abused. The book acknowledges too the plight of men who are trapped within a violent and abusive relationship and who also live in fear.

Finally, on behalf of these persons I would make a plea to all of you reading this no matter your role, your gender, your organization or your personal beliefs, if you can make a difference please endeavour to do so for no one is immune from abuse.

Contents

Appendices

Acknowledgements

I would like to thank Routledge for the opportunity to fulfil a long-time ambition, the chance to hopefully make a difference by supporting my healthcare colleagues to recognize and deal with the numerous clients that seek help to combat the effects of domestic abuse.

My gratitude to Dr Dawn Hillier, Dean of Health Care Practice, for her support and guidance; to Professor Gina Wisker for her patience when other deadlines were delayed in order that I could focus on writing the book; to Professor Colin Harrison who funded the writing of my first open learning package in domestic violence; to the students who have undertaken my Domestic Abuse modules, and even now are making an impact in midwifery practice and within other clinical settings; and to those colleagues in Health Care Practice, and in the University Centre for Learning and Teaching, who have helped to keep me resolute, you know who you are.

In particular I would like to thank my colleagues, and now my friends, Jean Flint, Catherine Wright, Hazel Taylor and Sharon Waller for their continuing friendship, humour, insight and support; Andrew Wood and Maurice Crockard for their fortitude, for their words of wisdom and for lending a listening ear; and to my colleagues in Ashby House who never fail to keep me grounded. I would like to acknowledge the work undertaken by Victim Support Essex and the opportunity they give me to continue to work with individuals who experience abuse and violence at the hands of an intimate partner.

In addition, to my son-in-law Jason, to my family in Wales, and to my friends, thank-you for being there. To my friends Marilyn Fenner and Jo Colling, a special thank-you for your unwavering faith in my ability to complete the project and to do it well.

I would like to acknowledge the individuals and organizations that have allowed me to draw upon their expertise in the subject with particular thanks to those whose work has been reproduced within the text and the appendices. Especial thanks to Women's Aid Federation of England, Newham Domestic Violence Forum, and Dr Iona Heath from the Royal College of General Practitioners. Crown Copyright material is produced with permission of the Controller of HMSO and the Queen's Printer for Scotland.

Never has there been a better time to act to curtail violence and abuse in the home. We therefore offer our gratitude and admiration to the women who have worked so tirelessly and with such passion and dedication over the past decades to bring today's practitioners in the field to the point where our work in this area is now possible and will in time become mainstream.

Chapter 1

Domestic violence – a healthcare issue

For many women and their families the effects of domestic violence will be catastrophic, the damage to their physical and psychological well being may be deeply damaging, and on occasions fatal.

(Department of Health [DoH] 2000a: 12)

DEFINING DOMESTIC VIOLENCE

Domestic violence has been defined as:

a continuum of behaviour ranging from verbal abuse, physical, and sexual assault, to rape and even homicide. The vast majority of such violence, and the most severe and chronic incidents, are perpetrated by men against women and their children.

(Department of Health [DoH] 2000a: v)

While the term 'domestic violence' includes violence and abuse within same-sex relationships, violence by women against men and violence and abuse perpetrated by one family member against another, the focus of this book is on violence and abuse by men, against women. It seeks to explore the multiplicity of factors that collectively construct an ever-increasing and serious healthcare need for those being abused within their intimate relationships.

Intimate violence may take many forms, often combining physical, emotional, psychological, sexual and financial abuse. The degree of abuse and violence varies within each partnership, often occurring on a continuum of severity and effect. For some the abuse and violence are periodic with minimal long-term effects. However, countless women are so controlled and inhibited that they are unable to make even the simplest decision or act without permission, responding with complete obedience to every order given and every rule imposed. The violence becomes insidious, permeating every action, every thought and deed until eventually, for some women, suicide remains the only escape. Other women express their self-disgust and powerlessness through alcohol or drug abuse, or self-mutilation, exhibiting signs of severe depression and total dependency on the abuser. Intimate partners may demand and achieve, through physical and emotional violence, complete obedience to every order, using humiliation as an important strategy in obedience training in their women.

As stated above, abuse and violence may be physical, emotional, psychological, financial or sexual, may be constant or spasmodic, and are experienced by individuals from every class, race, religion and culture the world over (British Medical Association [BMA] 1999).

Key point

The content of this book focuses in the main on the abuse in an intimate relationship of a woman by the man with whom she is having, or has had, an intimate relationship. However, it is important to note that when designing and developing procedures and protocols to deal with incidents related to domestic violence, a gender-neutral definition may be more effective in practice. To focus entirely on the needs of heterosexual females excludes other women and men, leaving them at risk.

SOME OF THE FACTS AND FIGURES

One in four women experience violence in the home at least once during their lifetime.

(Women's Aid Federation of England 2002)

Statistics reveal that one in four women experience violence in the home at least once in their lives, whilst many are subjected to long-term violence and abuse (British Medical Association [BMA] 1999; Department of Health [DoH] 2000a; Frost 1999a).

DOMESTIC VIOLENCE AND ABUSE – A HEALTHCARE ISSUE?

Historically the plight of women who are abused has largely been ignored by the majority of healthcare practitioners, often owing to a lack of understanding of either the problem or the potential solutions. However, in the 1990s, alongside other public services such as the police service, social services and local authorities, healthcare practitioners have increasingly recognized that violence and abuse in the home is an important, if not urgent, collective issue. In 1996, the World Medical Association, having recognized that doctors have a major role to play in the prevention and treatment of family violence, recommended that national medical associations should encourage and enable research to understand the prevalence, risk factors, outcomes and care needs for those experiencing family violence.

The Department of Health (2000a) summarizes the way forward for healthcare practitioners as follows:

Whether in general practice, dentistry, health visiting, nursing, maternity services, psychiatry and mental healthcare, general medicine and surgery, or in Accident and Emergency care, healthcare practitioners have daily contact with patients whose health is damaged by domestic violence, and who often face risks of further

and more extreme injury. The NHS response must not be seen simply in terms of treating the consequences of abuse, without also addressing the underlying causes. This responsibility rests with all healthcare practitioners who have contact with patients including those who have an on-going relationship such as through General Practice, Health Visiting, or Midwifery, and those who may have only a fleeting contact with someone in crisis, such as in Accident and Emergency departments.
(Yvette Cooper, Parliamentary Under-Secretary of State for Public Health, the NHS Executive, foreword to Department of Health 2000)

Despite initiatives from the Department of Health (hereafter DoH in discursive text), the British Medical Association (hereafter BMA in discursive text), and professional nursing and midwifery and health visiting bodies, there is little evidence that the majority of healthcare practitioners can either distinguish or effectively manage care of clients presenting with health problems related to domestic violence (British Medical Association [BMA] 1999; Department of Health [DoH] 2000a: 2; Frost 1999a). However, in recent years important work related to domestic violence in health and social care has been accomplished by researchers and practitioners across the United Kingdom Much of this work is acknowledged in the ensuing chapters, and in the key resources in Appendix 1.

It is essential that all healthcare practitioners gain insight and expertise into the nature of domestic abuse including alternative explanations of the causes, contributory factors and local and national interventions. In this way, all levels of healthcare practitioners can unite with other professional and voluntary groups to provide a quality service which meets the needs of all those involved in abusive circumstances.

WHAT'S IN A NAME?

Historically the term 'battered woman', or 'battered wife', has been acceptable terminology, but more recently it has come to be viewed by many in the field as an inappropriate term.

'Battered' conjures up an image of a woman lying beaten and bleeding, possibly in a state of physical exhaustion, and often in need of medical intervention, whereas the reality is that injuries may well be hidden and the damage virtually undetectable to the naked eye. Growing evidence confirms that countless women live their lives in constant fear and degradation, suffering severe psychological and emotional abuse perhaps without the accompanying broken bones and bruises. The abuse may be incessant whilst the physical violence is only periodic, but the results remain the same, a woman is being abused and therefore violated (Mayhew et al. 1996).

Terminology becomes especially important when one considers the concerned professional on the alert for a 'battered' woman, looking for the signs of physical injury, unaware of the reality. It is not surprising, therefore, that the abuse of many women accessing health services with other injuries, conditions or related needs may go undetected. The term 'battered' ignores the significant and persistent psychological, sexual, emotional injury and financial deprivation experienced by many thousands of women on a daily basis for long periods of their lives. It is this type of abuse which may lead to mental illness and attempts at self-harm, including suicide attempts, and may never present in physical injury.

VICTIM OR SURVIVOR?

Continuing discourse relates to the use of the terms 'victim' and 'survivor'. Whilst the former term symbolizes a woman crushed, beaten, helpless and powerless, the term 'survivor' signifies one who has overcome, or is currently overcoming, adversity. It is argued that being seen by others or seeing oneself as a 'victim' exacerbates the sense of powerlessness and resignation to one's fate. It can also be argued that women who access healthcare services with injuries, or struggle with problems resulting from abuse, are in fact 'victims' of violence. However, where possible within this text the term 'victim' is avoided as it does little to move the discourse forward or serve the women we are endeavouring to support.

Women experiencing intimate violence and abuse are not a homogeneous group, neither are the men who abuse them. Therefore, one-dimensional accounts of cause and effect are manifestly inadequate if the care offered is to be of practical use. Understanding, for some, lies in explanations at the level of society as well as of the individual, whilst for others the cause lies within the pathology of the individual. To disregard the wider political and social construction of domestic abuse is detrimental to the care that can be offered to the client. To do so leads to the 'medicalization' of domestic violence which ultimately structures the actual and potential approaches to care (Abbott and Williamson 1999).

Key point

Healthcare practitioners need to acknowledge and accept that domestic violence has a multiplicity of causal relationships that can make survival on occasion impossible and intervention fraught with difficulty. To ignore this premise, may lead the healthcare practitioner to provide one-dimensional care in the belief that there is little else that can be done. Patching a woman's wounds and sending her on her way ought not to be an option.

DOMESTIC VIOLENCE AND ABUSE: THE SIZE OF THE PROBLEM

A hidden crime

Not only are domestic violence and abuse a hidden figure in the crime statistics, they are also concealed from friends, from family, from work colleagues and others. How do so many women live with abuse for years without ever speaking out? In 1983, a study by Hopayian revealed that 89 per cent of women in refuges had consulted their general practitioner (GP) but nearly half hid the fact that they were being abused. This raises the question of why so many abused women access healthcare services and yet so few are recognized as being abused (British Medical Association [BMA] 2000).

Whilst many abusive acts are abhorrent they are not always deemed to be criminal. Nevertheless, domestic violence accounted for one-quarter of all violent crimes shown in the 1996 British Crime Survey (BCS). This is explored in further detail later in the chapter. Historically, even when women spoke out and reported violence, police responding to domestic incidents did little to intervene unless they absolutely had to. Today the police service is playing an important and changing role in addressing domestic violence and this will be explained in more detail in Chapter 8.

Violence against women is a crime: some of the statistics

> In the United Kingdom, two women every week are killed by a man with whom they have had, or are having an intimate relationship.
>
> (Home Office 2001a)

Statistics related to domestic violence must always be viewed with caution. Apart from rapes and sexual assault, the hidden crime figure for domestic violence is probably larger than for any other category of crime. For various reasons, either the crime is not reported to the police or, alternatively, it is not recorded and thus statistics related to the prevalence and nature of domestic violence are dependent upon who is collecting the data (Dobash et al. 1996; Home Office 2000a; Stanko 1998).

Mullender (1996), summarizing the debate on criminal statistics related to domestic violence, acknowledged that only from two to 27 per cent of incidents are reported to the police. She emphasizes that the 'constant terrorizing that goes on between each assault is equally a part of living with male abuse, but is not measurable in the same way'. Exploring the dilemma of how to quantify the magnitude of domestic abuse, Mooney (2000: 25), states that: 'levels of non-reporting are thought to be considerable for various reasons: fear of reprisals (the perpetrator may be near to the interview situation), embarrassment, psychological blocking and so on'. These findings are not dissimilar to an earlier study undertaken by Walklate in 1989. Walby and Myhill (2000: 1) acknowledge that current statistics related to violence against women generally are limited, as they use a relatively narrow definition of violence and do not include women outside of the home.

Furthermore, as domestic violence is recorded only in terms of physical and/or sexual assault, the numerous women subjected to emotional and psychological abuse almost certainly do not appear within criminal, social, or healthcare statistics. Mooney warns that the on-going paucity of substantive statistics on domestic violence in effect limits the ability to take appropriate preventative and remedial action. More realistic data, according to Mooney (2000), has been collected as a result of victimization studies such as that carried out by Mirlees-Black et al. (1999) and Mooney (1993).

Various studies have identified the reasons for under-reporting. These include:

- fear of further or escalating violence should the victim report an incident
- hopes that the relationship can be salvaged
- mistrust of agencies
- lack of knowledge about what most agencies could do to help.

Measures to identify victims of domestic violence form an important part of any domestic violence strategy. Studies highlight the importance of equipping workers in a range of agencies to detect domestic violence and take appropriate follow-up action, both through training (including multi-agency training) and through developing protocols (Mooney 2000).

Statistics from the United Kingdom

> The incidence of all categories of violence has increased since 1981, particularly domestic violence (240 per cent) and that by acquaintances (120 per cent).
>
> (Shepherd 1998)

In 1992 the British Crime Survey reported that 11 per cent of women living with their partner experienced some degree of physical violence within their relationship. Later, in 1996, the British Crime Survey (Mirrlees-Black 1999) provided what is probably the best available data for domestic violence in England and Wales (Walby and Mayhill 2000) showing that:

- At least one in four women in the UK experience varying degrees of violent assaults from an intimate partner, at some point during their life. (Many of course endure it for a significant part of that life.)
- Domestic violence accounts for one-quarter of all violent crimes reported in England.
- Criminal statistics for England and Wales (1997) showed that 47 per cent of female homicide victims were killed by their partners (compared to eight per cent of men). In real terms this means that every week at least two women are killed by their current or former partner (Home Office 2000a). Women are far more likely to be injured in the home by a partner than they are to fall victim to a stranger-crime.
- The study also found that women aged between 16 and 29 are at greatest risk of experiencing domestic violence, one reason perhaps why there is a growing focus on exploring violence in dating relationships.
- Women who separate from their partners more commonly suffer violence than women in other marital statuses. The study demonstrated that 22 per cent of separated women were assaulted by their partners or ex-partners.
- The incidence of all categories of violence has increased since 1981, particularly domestic violence (240 per cent) and that by acquaintances (120 per cent) (Shepherd 2001).
- On average, a woman is beaten at least 34 times before she seeks help.
- The highest incidence of domestic violence was reported by women aged between 20 and 24. Of these [i.e. the women aged 20–24] 28 per cent had experienced assault.

According to Shepherd (2001) what is important in a medical context, is the phenomenon of repeat victimization which is more common for violence than for other crimes:

- Of victims in the 1995 British Crime Survey, 30 per cent (and 43 per cent in a 1989 Accident and Emergency department survey [Shepherd 1990]) had been assaulted before by a current or ex-partner.
- Fear of reprisals and a continuing relationship with the assailant prevent men as well as women from reporting offences (Clarkson et al. 1994).

Walby and Myhill (2000) undertook an analysis for the Home Office to establish predisposing factors to domestic violence and their findings supported the above statistics. They further suggested, not surprisingly, that: 'Egalitarian partnerships have lower risk of domestic violence. The risk is increased by marital dependency and lack of economic resources. Unemployed women or housewives had a higher risk of domestic violence' (2000: n.p.).

Key point

There is a need for staff in healthcare departments to establish and maintain effective methods of collecting and recording data. This data must relate to assessing the client's needs; the incident; methods of intervention; and evaluation of strategies used for clients presenting with healthcare needs as a consequence of domestic abuse.

Domestic violence and murder

In early 2002, the Home Office acknowledged that at least two women in England and Wales are brutally murdered each week by an existing or past partner. Statistics published by the Metropolitan Police Service (MPS) highlighted that in the year 2001 there had been 36 domestic violence murders in the capital alone, a total of 25 per cent of all murders in this police district. Extrapolated nationally this figure indicates that approximately 35 per cent of all murders are linked to domestic violence.

In the last 10 years, police services across Great Britain have designed and implemented progressive policies and procedures related to the handling of domestic violence incidents. For example, in December 2000, the MPS launched a pro-active strategy called 'Enough is Enough' to demonstrate their commitment to dealing with all reported incidents of domestic violence. Police services all over the country have continued to develop and improve the service offered to victims of violence within the home.

AN INTERNATIONAL PERSPECTIVE ON VIOLENCE AGAINST WOMEN

It is important to recognize that violence against women is an international reality, only recently acknowledged as a major public health issue. Women's rights in many countries across Europe and the rest of the world remain either non-existent or embedded in archaic laws. Therefore, violence against women, particularly within the home, is often uncategorized, poorly defined, unrecorded, or seriously under-reported, resulting in either poor or non-existent services for abused women.

For example:

- In Germany, the results of victimization surveys are not even included in crime data-collection systems, despite the fact 40,000 women annually seek refuge in women's shelters.
- Similarly no official national data is kept in Thailand, Russia, or Italy.
- Only recently, after international pressure, has Japan acknowledged that a man does not have the right to use physical violence to chastise his wife. Subsequently, it is estimated that as a result over 11,000 Japanese women annually now cite violence as a reason for applying for divorce.

- Recently in six Australian jurisdictions there were 3,000 cases of domestic violence over one month.
- In South Africa, it is estimated that half of the reported sex offences and assaults on women, occur in private homes.
- In Jamaica, domestic violence is recognized as a major social problem. In Kingston alone there are approximately 900 murders annually of which 34 per cent occur in a domestic context.

(Summers and Hoffman 2002: xv)

In addition, Huch (2000), summarizing international studies, found that:

- In 1998, 66.7 per cent of the surveyed women in Sierra Leone had experienced physical abuse at the hands of their partners.
- In 1997 in the Middle East, 32 per cent of women reported being physically abused during the past year.
- A study undertaken in the Kissi district in Kenya in 1990 reported that 58 per cent of women said they were beaten often or sometimes.

Additional data on international statistics, from the *Watchtower*, November 2001, acknowledged that:

- In one year, 14,500 Russian women were killed by their husbands, and a further 56,400 were disabled or badly injured in domestic attacks.' (*Guardian*)
- Hong Kong: 'The number of women who say they have been beaten by their partners has soared by more than 40 per cent in the past year.' (*South China Morning Post*, 21 July 2000)
- Japan: The number of women seeking shelter rose from 4,843 in 1995 to 6,340 in 1998. 'About one-third said they were seeking shelter because of violent behaviour by their husbands.' (*Japan Times*, 10 September 2000)

Moreover, women in many countries are still subjected to violence in other ways such as:

- sex-selection abortion of a female foetus, often forced
- female infanticide, again often against the mother's wishes
- female genital mutilation of young girls
- incest, not designated illegal
- marital rape.

WHY DO MEN ABUSE WOMEN?

Conceivably, one explanation to the question why does a man batter and abuse his female partner is – because he can. It is beyond belief, but nevertheless true, that in the twenty-first century, there are some men who still believe in their right to chastise their female partner, even though they themselves may not have used violence against their partner.

FEMINIST PERSPECTIVE ON DOMESTIC ABUSE

Historical role of men

Within a social milieu advocating a 'return to family values' lies an assumption that the 'traditional' two-gender, two-parent family is conducive to individual, family and societal well-being. Yet, only a few decades ago a man was within his legal right to beat his wife using a reasonable degree of chastisement and not until the 1960s was marital rape recognized in law. For those wishing to extend their knowledge in this particular area, Atkins and Hoggett (1984) give a brief but comprehensive history of what they call 'the bread-winner's legal authority' which they maintain still existed in the courts in the 1980s.

According to Hague and Malos (1998: 57), the traditional male and female roles in relationships continue to exist in many homes today, with the man determining the 'rules' of the house, and the woman acknowledging his right to do so. They report on a study carried out in Islington by Middlesex University, in which only 37 per cent of the men surveyed did *not* see violence as an option, with 19 per cent admitting to violence against their female partner. If this is the 'hidden figure' of domestic violence then the reality is one that does not bear thinking about.

As recently as 1995, Joseph McGrail was found guilty of the manslaughter of his female partner and was given a suspended sentence because, according to the judge, he was provoked. Provocation includes: the female nagging, being unfaithful, failing in her domestic duties, etc. (Mullender 1996: 47). There exists an abundance of evidence clearly showing that for many women the world over, equality remains a delusion, and violence and abuse within the home a daily reality.

Women coexist with men in a society dominated by men, with legal and social norms historically defined, defended, and maintained by powerful men (Dobash and Dobash 1992; Hanmer and Itzen 2000). This is never more evident than when one explores the history of police intervention in family violence. Women have campaigned at length to convince those in the justice system that an assault occurring within the home is as illegal as one taking place in a public place, and therefore requires similar interventions and consequences.

Gaudoin (2001: 26) reporting on domestic violence identified that:

> One of the biggest problems to overcome where domestic violence is concerned is gender inequality. In a country where most of the law-makers, law enforcement officials and policy-makers are still men, getting society to recognize that a high proportion of its male population is dangerous inside the home was never going to be easy. Feminism was, and is, an easy target.

Feminist authors often highlight the continuing dependence of women upon men for financial support, despite the introduction of direct payment to women of the family allowance in the 1970s. Even a working woman sharing her home with a male partner may not be financially independent and may not therefore be in a position to leave a violent home. Feminist authors and researchers differ significantly on where they locate the origins of domestic violence. Nevertheless, most agree that domestic violence and abuse arise out of the power and control men exercise over women, and from the unequal position of women in society (Hague and Malos 1998: 58–9).

In subsequent chapters, it is noted how women are often trapped within an abusive relationship because they have limited access to adequate, alternative housing, financial support, legal services, and a safe environment in which to live.

> The economic and power relations are very different when one is considering domestic violence against a middle class but financially dependent wife, as compared to domestic violence against a single mother of three living in a local authority flat, or violence against a professional woman.
>
> (Mama 1996: 46)

In recent years studies seeking to explain male violence generally, and towards the female partner specifically, have been undertaken. One of the important findings to emerge is that men and women often have totally different perspectives as to what constitutes violent behaviour.

Perceptions of violence

In 1993, Mooney undertook a survey of 1,000 people in a North London borough, which included 571 women and 429 men. The survey showed that a clear majority of all women defined five main aspects of behaviour as domestic violence:

- mental cruelty
- threats
- physical violence without actual bodily harm
- physical violence with actual bodily harm
- being made to have sex without consent.

Men's views on their violence towards known women

In contrast, studies that have sought to clarify men's characterization of abuse suggest they typically only include extreme physical acts of violence. In Hearn's study (1996), women recurrently included shouting, swearing, abusive name-calling, threats of violence, slapping, throwing objects, and/or pushing, whereas most of the men only referred to extreme physical acts which caused obvious harm to the woman's body.

The Domestic Abuse Intervention Project (DAIP) in Duluth, Minnesota (hereafter referred to as the Duluth model) is one of the longest-running multi-agency projects working to change the behaviours of abusive perpetrators. Women who had been, or were being, abused, collectively identified those actions that they deemed to be abusive behaviour (Fig. 1, Duluth model of violent behaviour). The wheel model demonstrates the wide range of abusive behaviours used by men to control their female partners, including: physical and sexual assault; coercion and threats; intimidation; emotional abuse; social isolation; using male privilege; minimizing or denying behaviour; and economic sanctions.

Violence as an individual pathological condition

Pathological perspectives of violent and abusive behaviour seek to explain the phenomena at the level of the individual perpetrator or indeed the 'victim'. Such perspectives search

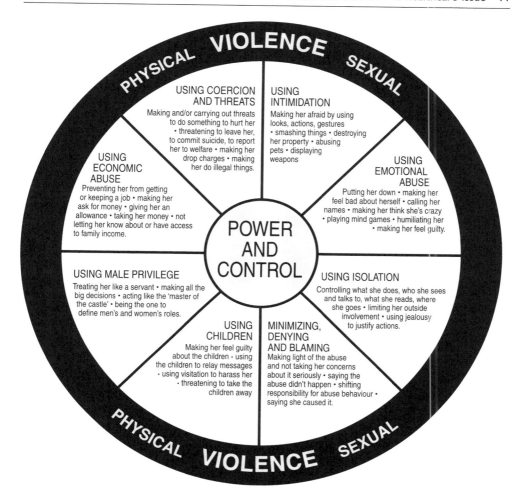

Figure 1 Duluth model of power and control. Reproduced with kind permission of the Minnesota Program Development, Inc.

for specific individual characteristics or situations that in certain individuals and/or circumstances instigate or contribute to a violent or abusive episode. For example, studies have confirmed that perpetrators of violence in the home or in the community may be under the influence of, and sometimes addicted to, alcohol and/or illegal substances (British Medical Association [BMA] 1999: 23). However, such explanations have their limitations, as many men who misuse alcohol and illegal substances do not resort to abusing their female partners.

In challenging the notion that excessive use of alcohol and drugs causes a predisposition to domestic violence, Mullender (1996: 34), cites a 1980s' study undertaken by Kantor and Strauss. Their study established that 80 per cent of 'heavy'- and 'binge'-drinking men did not hit their female partners during the twelve months of the survey. Moreover,

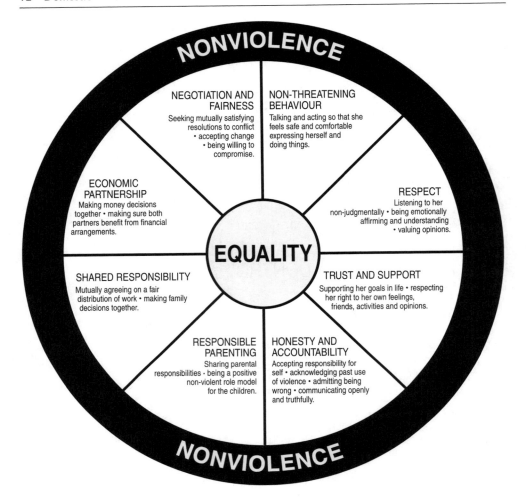

Figure 2 Duluth model of equality. Reproduced with kind permission of the Minnesota Program Development, Inc.

McGibbon and Kelly's study (1989: 32), cited in Mullender (1996: 34), confirmed that men drank before abusing women to give themselves 'Dutch' courage. The drinking gives them 'permission' to be violent, or provides an excuse to call upon after the event. The abuser who can excuse his behaviour in this way is apt to gain forgiveness from his female partner, at least for a while. Similarly, alternative perspectives have identified specific traits said to be present in male abusers, such as addictive personalities, mental illness, and excessive aggressive tendencies. Dobash and Dobash (1992: 237) identified contemporary psychological theories which support the notion of 'uncontrollable violent outbursts often located in unresolved family conflicts, primitive aggressive reactions, the submerged fear of the bully, insecure dependence on women, or any other form of internal stress'.

One of the counter-arguments to this perspective is that these men most often direct their 'uncontrollable violence' at women with whom they are having an intimate relationship rather than the world at large. They abuse those least given to fighting back or those least in a position to cause physical harm to the aggressor. Were the violence 'uncontrollable' it would erupt more frequently and to a wider group of individuals or groups; equally there are men who own up to having outbursts of anger but would never hit their female partner. This is particularly relevant if a member of the health team is considering recommending or sending an abusive man on to an 'anger management' programme (Taylor-Browne 2001: 64). (A more detailed examination of anger-management and other forms of intervention is discussed later in the book.) Such findings were confirmed in a study by Ptacek (1988), when 17 out of the 18 men in a group trying to deal with their abusive behaviour claimed 'loss of control'. However, only 5 of these men were violent outside, as well as inside, the home. In Ptacek's work, the men stated that the reasons they abused their female partner was because they wanted to frighten and hurt her, because she provoked them and because she hadn't been a good wife. Some of the men interviewed admitted that they were often able to control the degree and type of violence, but insisted that when they did not control it, they were blameless.

Theories associated with 'uncontrollable violence' do not adequately explain men who supplement their outbursts of 'sudden rage' with systematic psychological abuse, including constantly demeaning their partner in public, financial abuse, sexual abuse, and (if the woman leaves) stalking, making threatening phone calls and even murdering her. Equally, there have been attempts to typify the 'abused woman' as one who is submissive, frail, mentally and spiritually weak, etc. Whilst there is evidence that a proportion of women over time exhibit such attitudes and behaviour, there is little if any evidence to sustain the belief that the 'abused women' have always been like this.

On the contrary, women who are being abused may have jobs and careers; be employed in positions of power; make important business decisions; and be viewed by the outside world as successful career women. Yet, in the world they call their home they are subjected to abuse on a daily basis. Women may experience continuous attempts to undermine their self-esteem, their inherent worth, and then as they leave their homes to go to work don a completely different mantle. In fact, the Islington study showed that 25 per cent of professional women reported having been abused compared to 30 per cent of working-class women. However, professional women report the violence to the police or other agencies less frequently, but are more likely to tell friends and family (Mooney 1994).

Henwood (2000) suggests that professional women seek external intervention less frequently because they have independent resources and the option to make choices without recourse to statutory services. This assumes that professional women are more financially and emotionally independent than their counterparts from the working classes. The Home Office study (Walby and Myhill 2000) also identified similar proportions of professional and working-class males that admitted to hitting their partners.

Key points

Abused women come from many diverse worlds, different social classes, cultures, and ethnic groups, and all experience their abusive relationship in quite a different way. Consequently, there can be no one-dimensional explanation of cause and effect, and the healthcare practitioners must put aside their personal beliefs and prejudices if they are to offer appropriate care and support. All healthcare practitioners need to gain an insight into the different aspects of domestic violence and abuse. Only then will they be in a position to assess, plan, implement, and evaluate effective evidence-based care, of all abused persons.

Whilst not dismissing the prospect that those responsible for violence and abuse within relationships may have a pathological condition, such an explanation alone is inadequate. One must question why others with similar characteristics do not behave in a violent or abusive way towards their partners.

A biological explanation of violence

Scientists have endeavoured to locate male violence within a biological framework, arguing that anger and thus violence is an innate instinct, genetically determined and therefore often not under the control of the individual perpetrator. This implies that men's aggression and their violence against women are in some way at least understandable, if not justifiable. If we accept such a stance, how then do we explain women who also appear to behave with extreme, seemingly uncontrolled, violence in certain circumstances? Conversely, if we dismiss such explanations are we not also dismissing the growing literature which suggests that there is a correlation between female reproductive hormones, depression and feelings of anger in women, i.e. pre-menstrual syndrome (PMS)?

Violence as learned behaviour

> Human beings always have choices (and hence responsibilities for their behaviour); we are not pre-programmed like a machine. Indeed people who have lived with abuse may have more motivation for avoiding it later in life since they have seen the damage it can inflict.
>
> (Mullender 1996: 40)

Alternative theories propose that adult violence is learned behaviour, the result of an abusive childhood in which the emerging adult either becomes an abuser or remains a victim long into adulthood. Consequently, children suffering at the hands of a violent parent carry that experience forward into adulthood, thus continuing the cycle of violence for many generations (Hague and Malos 1998: 53).

Such explanations may gain credibility, especially with the wider public, as they create and sustain a myth that somehow domestic violence occurs within deviant families thus reassuring the average man and woman that it does not happen to them (Hague and

Malos 1998: 53). Others, however, challenge these beliefs, maintaining that significant numbers of children from violent homes develop into non-violent adults.

Equally there exists a strong therapeutic culture, including neo-Freudianism and many forms of psychotherapy, based on the premise that psychological problems in adulthood have their origins in a dysfunctional childhood and adolescence. Wilson (1983), whilst supporting an inter-generational explanation, argues that although it may have credence for explaining violence within some relationships it is a deficient theory for the whole. The short- and long-term effects on children living in a violent home are explored in detail in Chapter 2.

DOES IT MATTER HOW WE DEFINE IT?

Adopting a particular theoretical stance determines where one locates the cause of the problem and therefore where the focus of intervention lies. For example, if domestic violence is a result of an individual deviance or inadequacy, there is no need for society at large to make major changes to its structures and functions. In this instance, the solution to the problem might lie in setting up treatment centres for the violators, offering them aggression management therapy, and at the same time supporting the women through assertiveness training and therapy. Whereas such interventions may transform a range of individuals, or advantage some couples, offering them as a major solution does not acknowledge the complex and multi-dimensional elements often present in violent relationships. Conversely, if the problem is located solely at the level of society or the culture within which we live, the inference is that an individual within that society is relatively powerless to effect change and the status quo will continue.

Key point

Whatever the research shows, and whatever the experts offer as explanations for violence and abuse within intimate relationships the healthcare practitioner should never forget that:

> Given that the pattern of domestic violence is one of escalation, there is no level of abuse which should be viewed, as acceptable or insignificant. Indeed intervening at an early stage has the potential to prevent the abuse escalating.
>
> (Henwood 2000: 9)

DATING VIOLENCE AS A SOCIAL PHENOMENON

Dating violence may be defined as the perpetration or threat of an act of violence by at least one member of an unmarried couple on the other member within the context of dating or courtship. This violence encompasses any form of sexual assault, physical violence, and verbal or emotional abuse.

(National Center for Injury Prevention and Control, January 2000)

This section focuses primarily on 'dating violence' between young people, as the issues for older couples dating are similar to those already covered elsewhere. In recent years, literature on violence amongst young people in intimate relationships, and what has become known as 'dating violence', has increased exponentially, as it seems has 'date rape' across a spectrum of age groups.

The National Center for Injury Prevention and Control (January 2000) summarizing past and recent studies, identified that prevalence rates of non-sexual, courtship violence ranged from nine per cent to 65 per cent, depending on whether threats and emotional or verbal aggression were included in the definition. Generally, the violence was non-sexual although the amount of sexual violence increased according to age groups, with female undergraduate students reporting the most sexual assaults. Figures from the United Kingdom are to date limited, although the ESRC study undertaken by staff from the University of Warwick in the UK found that:

> Over 75 per cent of 11–12 year old boys thought that women get hit if they make men angry, and more boys than girls, of all ages, believed that some women deserve to be hit. Boys aged 13–14 were less clear that men should take responsibility for their violence. Boys of all ages, particularly teenagers, have less understanding than girls of who is at fault, and are more likely to excuse the perpetrator.
>
> (Mullender 2000: n.p.)

Such facts are liable to be significant when translated into teen and young adult dating relationship.

Römkens and Mastenbroek (1998) in summarizing recent international studies concluded that insufficient research has yet been done on the existence, impact, or consequences of violence between young dating couples. Similarly, they acknowledged that more work is required into dating violence of a sexual nature across all age groups within an intimate dating relationship. Römkens and Mastenbroek (1998: 59) describe a violent or abusive dating relationship, as one in which there is a 'rapid alternation between romantic expectations and hope, on the one hand and shame and fascination, on the other'. The young woman is often left confused and increasingly socially isolated as she chooses not to share the experience with close friends or family. Ferguson (1998: 84) undertakes to identify and critique existing studies in this area, and highlights the need for more systematic recording and explorations of this area of behaviour. Her work concludes that relationship violence between young people is a serious public health issue worthy of further work. According to Berry (2000), some experts have estimated that 'dating violence' occurs in between 20 to 30 per cent of adolescent relationships.

The debates in the area of 'dating violence' appear to be very similar to those of intimate violence as we will explore it in this book. To date there is no agreed definition, no systematic way to assess, manage, or evaluate intervention strategies. Similarly, there is no consensus as to how the problems related to dating violence might be tackled, although most writers appear to agree that not only is it a serious health and social problem, but often the psychological and physical abuse escalates into sexual abuse and assault.

Ferguson (1998: 98) summarizes previous research into adolescent dating violence as identifying the following characteristics:

- The relationship is often based on historic gender differentiation roles. Consequently, young women take responsibility for the success or otherwise of the relationship. Referring to the early work of Dobash and Dobash, published in 1989, and of Levy, published in 1991 and 1993, Ferguson suggests that the young woman is in all probability socially dependent upon the male, and accedes to his demands for her undivided attention. She may even perceive this to be a sign of his devotion.
- It is possible that she is required to surrender social activities which do not include him, including going out with her girlfriends, groups she may belong to, etc.
- Again, the male is apt to exhibit the sexist male pose, dictating what the female does, when and with whom.
- Acts of jealousy, aggression, or possessiveness are often viewed by the young woman as romantic expressions of the male's devotion.

Other studies indicate that the young woman may be isolated from her family, or no longer influenced by their views. Therefore, when the situation escalates to more serious physical or sexual violence, she may not feel able to seek help from them. Alternatively, some studies show that the family might underestimate the seriousness of what the young woman is saying.

Young women particularly at risk of becoming trapped in abusive relationships include those from ethnic minority groups, as dating an 'outsider' may have already caused them problems with the family. Young men and women in gay relationships may be vulnerable because 'confusion about norms and roles may be acted out in a relationship' (Ferguson 1998: 99). Berry (2000) suggests that adolescents in an abusive relationship may find exiting particularly challenging as they may not have sufficient knowledge to know what options are available. She suggests that young people may find those that could help, such as parents, teachers, and police, intimidating or unlikely to take it seriously. One also has to acknowledge that adolescence is a period of exploration and of discovery. Therefore, many teenagers may not appreciate that this is not 'normal' dating behaviour, especially if their own childhood experience has been marred by violence.

Young people's self-esteem is especially vulnerable and fragile, with peer approval being so vital to one's self-worth. Therefore, it is a time when the young woman 'wants to be like everyone else', she wants to be in a 'loving' relationship. She is apt to take the blame more easily than an older woman and neither does she have the perspective and experience of an older woman. 'Young women tend to be susceptible to romantic notions that "true love" means an all encompassing passion that allows for jealousy, possessiveness, and aggression as a demonstration of devotion and commitment' (Berry 2000: 141).

It is perhaps interesting to note that in the last few years, men who would normally be viewed as 'super-heroes', romantic figures for young women, have been exposed in public for their violent or abusive behaviour. Today, it is not unusual to read of well-known footballers appearing in court for assaulting members of the public; film stars identified as wife-abusers; famous sportsmen exposed as 'wife-beaters'; and even politicians having their personal conduct scrutinized by the public, and found wanting. What may have traditionally been viewed as 'normal behaviour for rock and pop stars' has been condemned as socially unacceptable, as have musical lyrics advocating anti-social behaviour. Historically this behaviour might have been categorized as 'boys will be boys' or excused either because they were famous, or because they were under stress due to their fame. In contrast, more female public figures are divulging their personal experiences of violence and abuse in the hope that other women are influenced, and thus find the strength to leave their abusive partners. Well-known female singers, athletes, film and TV stars or wives of famous men have come forward to share their own journeys to recovery, often supporting national campaigns and women's organizations.

Key point

As healthcare providers, we have to ensure that the message that violence is intolerable, no matter the circumstances, is conveyed to as wide a public as possible. Policies and protocols related to abuse and violence must identify the specific needs of adolescents and young women as well as other very vulnerable groups of society.

Young women may not relate to generic materials written for women in intimate relationships. Therefore, materials written specifically for different user groups are essential if each individual is to feel that her circumstances are recognized and valued by the professional or helping agency. Equally, any public health campaigns for domestic violence should address the needs of all vulnerable groups wherever possible; for example, adverts specific to young women could be designed for publication in 'teen magazines'.

'DATE (OR ACQUAINTANCE) RAPE'

In recent years, there have been numerous reports internationally on what has generally become known as 'date or acquaintance rape', that is, sexual assault by a man upon a woman with whom he has a dating relationship. More recently, this definition has become connected to rape events in which the couples are not necessarily in short-term or long-term relationships, but may have simply 'dated' once or twice.

Römkens and Mastenbroek's (1998) study of 457 female Dutch students found that almost 19 per cent claimed to have had non-consensual sexual contact at some time with the person they were going out with.

> Since sex between adolescents and youngsters is inevitably a matter of uncertainty and ambivalence, exploring one another's boundaries and sexual desires is an activity in which things can indeed go wrong. . . . However they [the statistics] convincingly demonstrate that date rape is by no means exceptional.
>
> (Römkens and Mastenbroek 1998: 61)

As we saw above, rape in the UK is a common crime with a conviction rate of below 10 per cent and sentences as low as 180 hours community service. Between 1996 and 1997 the number of women reporting rape increased by over 500 per cent. Yet convictions have remained almost static, meaning that whilst in 1977, one in three women reporting rape saw their rapists convicted, in 1996 less than one in ten did. The criminal justice system is currently failing women, not just those who report rape, but every woman, since the message being sent out is that rape is a low-risk, high-reward activity. As we have already seen, the conviction rate for rape cases where the man and the woman are known to each other is even lower, especially in cases often known as date rape. In these circumstances there is almost no chance at all that the case reaches the court or if it does that the prosecution is successful.

CONCLUSION

If women, other vulnerable adults and children are to be protected from harm from current or previous partners then all members of the health services have an important role to play. Accessing health services may be the only opportunity the victims of abuse have to confide in someone with the knowledge and expertise to assist them in a manner that does not lead to further harm. There are countless reasons why abused individuals attending their GP surgery, hospital or local clinic do not disclose the violence and abuse they are enduring. These include shame, stigma, fear that their partner might find out that they have told someone or fear that their children may be taken into care. Often they may worry that the doctor, nurse, midwife, or health visitor may judge and despise them for continuing to stay within the relationship.

Every week in the United Kingdom women and men are dying at the hands of adults who profess love and devotion, whilst systematically abusing and violating them. It may be that the one time they access one of the health services may be their first and last chance to break the cycle of violence.

Key point

For this reason, all healthcare practitioners must:

- Challenge their own preconceptions of domestic violence in order that they can offer support in a professional and non-judgemental way.
- Be aware of the issues related to domestic violence and abuse, recognizing the signs that an individual is being abused.
- Accept that a lack of bruises and physical injury does not mean abuse is not occurring.
- Have either the requisite skills to assist the individual, or the knowledge of whom and where to refer them to.
- Create an environment which encourages disclosure by those experiencing the abuse.
- Advocate for appropriate systems and support within their work area.
- Have sufficient knowledge and expertise to offer evidence-based care to all those who are suffering from violence within their home, or from a partner who has recently left.
- Work, wherever possible, with people from other agencies so that collectively we can make a difference.

Chapter 2

The impact of domestic abuse on health

> Domestic violence has considerable implications for the NHS – particularly in Accident and Emergency departments, primary care and in specialist settings such as maternity services and child and adolescent mental health services. Healthcare costs are considerable; personal costs even more so – perhaps, especially if not acknowledged or recognized.
>
> (Department of Health [DoH] 1997a: 23)

DOMESTIC VIOLENCE: THE ROLE OF HEALTHCARE PRACTITIONERS

Measuring the impact of domestic violence on health is problematical, if not impossible, and undoubtedly extends beyond the immediacy of physical injury. Growing evidence illustrates how women and children living within a violent and abusive relationship may experience lifelong, adverse, health consequences. Nevertheless, there is an increasing realization that appropriately educated and trained healthcare practitioners can perform a significant role in supporting family members within violent relationships (British Medical Association [BMA] 1999).

Key point

Whilst this book mainly focuses on men's violence against women, it should be remembered that violence in intimate partnerships occurs in same-sex relationships, and that women do abuse men, both physically and mentally. Therefore, the following sections could relate to abuse in any intimate relationship.

Virtually every woman in the United Kingdom uses the healthcare system at some point in her life, whether for care for herself or in the role of carer for children or elderly people, putting healthcare practitioners in a unique access position. Nevertheless, many of these women continue to hide the fact that they are being abused at home and perhaps more importantly may never be asked the question. Women who have been abused, access health services with short-, medium- and long-term healthcare needs. A woman may visit her GP's surgery on a regular basis with vague, indeterminate signs and symptoms. Equally, she may visit the Accident and Emergency department with severe bruising and broken bones, or following an episode of deliberate self-harm. It is the role of each healthcare practitioner to ensure that the means and the resolve to offer appropriate care are available, whatever the circumstances, in whichever arena the woman appears.

As far back as 1983, a study undertaken by Hopayian *et al.* revealed that 89 per cent of women in refuges had consulted their GP. However, almost half concealed the fact they were being battered, as they were ashamed, or were afraid their partners would find out, or because they felt the attitude of the doctor was less than helpful. Sadly, there is little evidence to suppose that the situation has greatly improved in today's healthcare arena.

DOMESTIC VIOLENCE AND HEALTHCARE: THE STATISTICS

In the 1990s, the quality and quantity of British research into domestic violence, as it relates to healthcare, increased significantly. However, we remain a long way from constructing an effective, consistent, evidence-based, national health and social care response to the problem.

Key points

Findings of the Hackney study undertaken by Stanko *et al.* (1997) identified:

- One in four incidents of domestic violence result in substantial physical injury.
- Out of 129 women surveyed in a GP surgery, 10 per cent had been knocked unconscious, and five per cent had sustained broken bones as a result of domestic violence.
- On average each woman reported having sustained at least four or more of these injuries.
- In Mooney's study of 1993, 27 per cent of women suffered physical injury; six per cent broken bones; eight per cent were detained in hospital.
- Only 25 per cent of women who do seek medical help for domestic injuries admit that the injuries were caused by partner violence (Dobash and Dobash 1979).
- Abused women are more often in touch with the health services than any other agency (Pahl 1995).

Despite these alarming figures, as we see later many women will not report the real cause of the injury, and healthcare practitioners all too often do not ask too many questions.

RECOGNIZING DOMESTIC ABUSE IN A HEALTHCARE SETTING

Categorizing the type and degree of health need may lead to adverse outcomes for these women if the healthcare practitioner simply focuses on one or more particular 'sign or symptom', thus medicalizing domestic violence. In order to ensure that the whole gamut of consequences is covered, an attempt will be made to identify as many presenting healthcare needs as possible.

Recognizing physical injury

There are a number of features which may alert us to the fact the client is being physically abused, including:

- The injuries are not consistent with the account of how they occurred.
- The woman has attended with similar injuries before.
- There are signs of old bruising, old scars or, in severe cases, old fractures.
- There are injuries at various stages of healing.
- Bite marks are a not uncommon feature of intimate violence.
- The bruising may be extensive with a range of injuries occurring simultaneously. The British Crime Survey (1996) showed that almost one-third of the women interviewed required medical attention, with 69 per cent of incidents leading to injury and 13 per cent resulting in broken bones.
- The bruises may occur in unusual places; for example, bruises on the inner thigh are rarely a result of accidental injury.
- Women more frequently have injuries to the breast, chest, and abdomen (Stark and Flitcraft 1996), including fractured ribs.
- Facial injuries are common, including broken noses, jaws, teeth and cheekbones, split lips.
- Signs of attempted strangling or asphyxiation may be present; this is a significant sign that the abuser is dangerous (Berry 2000).
- The woman may be pregnant or experiencing pains associated with premature labour.
- There may be signs of injurious sexual activity.
- Abused women more often have internal injuries than do accident victims (Burge 1989).
- The woman may present with a sexually transmitted disease.

Psychological and emotional abuse

As we have already identified, women who have been abused often say that the emotional and psychological abuse they experience is for them the most destructive element. Similarly, studies of abuse against men have intimated that the mental cruelty is often what is most difficult to endure. Once a woman has been beaten it is not difficult to see how subsequent threats of more beatings might be sufficient to achieve submissiveness. Psychological and emotional abuse includes those acts designed to control, intimidate, ensure compliance. It may comprise:

- constant threats of violence against the woman, the children, and pets
- constant ridicule about almost all aspects of the woman's self and her ability to undertake tasks effectively. Ridiculing her looks, dress sense, sexual worth, intelligence, parenting abilities, housekeeping, driving: the list is endless.
- expectation of total compliance within the home
- humiliation, especially in front of other people, including friends, family members, children, work colleagues and others
- social isolation from friends and family, including preventing the woman from going out unaccompanied. This may include prohibiting the woman from employment outside of the home.

- compelling the woman to account for her time throughout the day including: timing visits to the doctor, dentist, shops, picking up the children from school and other actitivities
- ensuring economic dependency (financial abuse)
- controlling the manner in which the woman dresses, behaves, interacts with others
- name calling, use of abusive terms often of a sexual nature designed to humiliate
- making her feel guilty, persuading her that if she were a 'better wife and mother' then he would not need to be abusive
- playing mind games
- making her think she is mentally unstable.

Other signs that the woman may be in an abusive relationship include the following:

- There may be a delay in seeking healthcare intervention for injuries.
- The woman may be lethargic, unable to account for the injuries or unwilling to give details.
- She may be quiet, withdrawn and reluctant to discuss the problem.
- The partner may stay by her side constantly.
- The woman may not attend for follow-up appointments.
- The woman may be under the influence of alcohol or drugs.

The woman may not appear in the least intimidated or downtrodden but that does not mean she is not being brutalized.

Observing the partnership dynamics

It may be that the woman attends for care on her own, but equally the partner may ensure that he remains by his partner's side for the whole consultation and treatment period. The healthcare practitioner should monitor for aspects of controlling behaviour: for example, the partner answering for the woman, his insistence that he remains in the room, his attempts to control her version of events. This may be represented as intense caring behaviour and a reluctance to leave the side of the client.

At this point, it is crucial to remember that violence occurs in same-sex relationships, and therefore care should be taken if discussing the situation with a 'concerned friend' in attendance. To ensure the client's safety, it is preferable to provide the opportunity to talk alone with the healthcare practitioner. Similarly, not all domestic abuse is male against female or occurring between intimate partners. The abuse might be female against male, sibling abuse, an adult or adolescent child against a parent, or elder abuse. Therefore, it is essential that the client is given the opportunity to talk to the healthcare practitioner in confidence.

Key point

Domestic violence and abuse is a complex, multi-faceted phenomenon. For intervention to be adequate and appropriate, the healthcare practitioner should refrain from making assumptions about the perpetrator, the victim, the injuries, or the circumstances surrounding the incident. An open mind is more likely to lead to safe, effective care.

MARITAL/PARTNER SEXUAL ASSAULT AND RAPE

> Women raped by acquaintances found the experience even more difficult to come to terms with than those raped by strangers. They felt betrayed – not just by the men but by their own judgement. It made them more fearful of men generally, since they no longer knew who to trust.
>
> (Lees in Hanmer and Itzen 2000: 63)

Sexual assault in intimate relationships is thought to be widespread (Whately 1993). It includes: forced sex, including anal, vaginal and oral penetration; the use of implements in assaulting the partner sexually; urinating on the partner; forced tying-up of the partner; forcing the partner to mimic or take part in pornography; and enforced prostitution, including forcing the woman to take part in sexual acts with acquaintances. (British Medical Association [BMA] 1999).

'A survey of 1000 women in city centres in North England found that 1 in 8 women reported having been raped by their husbands or partners' (Painter 1991 in Lees 2000: 60). Since the change in the law, it is now also possible to prosecute a male for having unlawful sexual intercourse with another male as the definition now includes anal penetration, whereas previously it was confined to vaginal penetration.

One must bear in mind that sexual assault and rape are rarely, if ever, about sexual gratification: they are about coercion and control. Within an intimate relationship, sexual assault or rape is more often the result of the man's need to dominate, humiliate and control the person he later professes to love and care for. Women for centuries have been viewed by society as 'belonging' to their husbands, with no legal right to self-determination once married. Not until the end of the nineteenth century was 'wife-beating' defined as a criminal act, and only recently has marital rape been recognized by the British justice system. Prior to 1991, the 'marital rape exclusion' clause deemed that there could be no rape in marriage and therefore the perpetrator was free from criminal prosecution (Lees 1997).

Even when a man is charged with the offence of rape, statistics reveal that the criminal prosecution service (CPS) is less prone to prosecute a rape case in which the couple are married or cohabiting. Equally, when a prosecution is successful the sentences for such cases are significantly less than those for rape by strangers (Lees 1997), despite the fact that marital/partner rape is seven times as common as stranger rape (Painter 1991). The literature indicates that the courts view sexual assault and rape against a known adult to be a less traumatic event than when committed by a stranger. This is contrary to how women describe their experiences. Painter (1991), after reviewing the literature, concluded that marital or partner rape:

- is no less traumatic than stranger rape
- is not shown by evidence to be any less violent or dangerous than stranger rape
- is viewed by the woman as a betrayal of trust as well as a criminal act, and therefore has a negative impact on her recovery
- has effects on survivors that can be lengthy and traumatic
- more often includes strangling as a means of overpowering the victim than stranger rapes (comparative study)

- involves injuries not necessarily less severe than those inflicted during stranger rape
- receives significantly lower sentences in the courts when a case is brought.

Finally as a consequence of rape the woman may conceive, thus she faces the additional trauma of an unplanned and possibly unwanted pregnancy in which her choices of action are severely limited.

Research indicates that twice as many women raped by a stranger said they feared for their life, possibly because a higher proportion of strangers threaten to harm or kill their victims. According to Lees 'marital rape and murder are forms of extreme coercion often fuelled by revenge at the woman daring to leave or planning to leave preceded by extreme possessiveness' (2000: 61).

Role of the healthcare practitioner dealing with a sexual assault

The role of the healthcare practitioner dealing with a woman who has been sexually assaulted or raped by an intimate partner depends upon a number of factors. If the woman presents, possibly at the GP's surgery, or at an Accident and Emergency department as a recent trauma patient, then the work of the healthcare practitioner should focus in the first instance on immediate physical care.

Key point

Rape and sexual assault are serious criminal offences; therefore preserving the evidence should be an important consideration when determining the required clinical intervention. Most local police services have specialized teams of professionals to deal with all such incidents, including a forensic medical examiner. The overall aim both for healthcare staff and for the police is to minimize the trauma of care after the event. Therefore staff need to be aware of protocols related to the assessment, management and clinical interventions required for victims of sexual assault, both female and male. It must also be remembered that the explicit wishes of the injured person must be paramount in any decisions made by the professionals.

A more detailed account of care is addressed in Chapter 6 related to clinical interventions.

Escalation of the violence

The MPS (2001) estimate that approximately three out of five victims of reported domestic rape had previously reported an incident of domestic violence to the police. Furthermore, it was estimated that the rise in severity of the incidents could be rapid. In a study undertaken between January 2001 and March 2001, the MPS established that more than a third of all domestic violence offenders were flagged as being either high- or very high-risk for re-offending.

> **Key point**
>
> Professionals in the field acknowledge that the most dangerous time for a woman in an abusive relationship is the point at which she tries to leave, or is successful in leaving.

The role of the legal professions is explored in more detail in Chapter 6.

WHY DOESN'T SHE LEAVE?

> The question 'Why doesn't she leave' is victim blaming in itself, both because it puts the onus on the woman to act, and because it is the question most commonly asked; it is rare in comparison for people to ask 'Why does he abuse?'
>
> (Mullender 1996: 54)

For those outwith an abusive relationship it may be impossible to understand why the woman does not leave. Indeed, many of the women who appear on television talk shows seem to be inextricably linked to, and emotionally dependent on, their abuser. Even when faced with the realization that the relationship is unlikely to change, often the woman still appears to be unable to remove herself from danger. Alternatively, the woman succeeds in leaving for a short period only to return later. The reasons why are complex and may never be fully understood, what health professionals must focus on is supporting the woman wherever, whenever and however they can.

'The psychological impact of domestic violence has been found to have parallels with the impact of torture and imprisonment on hostages' (Hester *et al.* 2000: 132). Graham, Rawlings and Rimini (1988), in seeking to explore and explain the behaviour of women in long-term abusive relationships, likened their experience to that of hostages in siege situations, a phenomenon identified as the 'Stockholm syndrome'. Through observation, they offered the premise that as a result of being in a life-threatening situation over a sustained period, women often exhibit certain behavioural and psychological responses to the situation, similar to those exhibited by hostages. The model seeks to show how extreme power imbalances between an abusive male and his abused female partner can lead to strong emotional bonding. Hester *et al.* (2000: 21) assert that such a model may be useful when attempting to understand why the woman stays or why, even when she has managed to leave an abusive and violent relationship, the woman may return.

The 'hostage' situation is of course created and sustained when the man ensures his partner is socially isolated, financially dependent, and punished with impunity for an infraction of the 'house rules'. The power differential is prolonged by continuous depreciation and humiliation of the woman in public and in private, reaffirming her low self-esteem and confirming her inability to fend for herself and her children. The man, through unpredictable episodes of violence, possible continuous threats of death interspersed with periods of kind and loving behaviour, with promises of a brighter future maintains the emotional hold he has over the woman (Hester *et al.* 2000: 22). Whilst this model offers a possible rational foundation for why some women stay, it nevertheless portrays the woman as passive with few, if any, alternatives and it therefore does not apply to many abusive relationships.

Key points

The healthcare practitioner must always keep in mind, that a domestic violence situation is inevitably a complex, dynamic and volatile occurrence. Simplistic explanations do not provide the long-term solutions necessary for the woman wishing to move from the position of victim to that of survivor.

It should always be remembered that for many women in a violent relationship, leaving is commonly a lengthy and painful journey rather than a single desperate act. A woman is most at risk of severe physical injury or death at the point of leaving the relationship or after she has done so (Metropolitan Police Service 2002).

Previously, theorists such as Walker (1984) endeavoured to explain women's perceived inability to leave in terms of 'learned helplessness'. Describing the domestic violence situation as cyclical, with periods of escalating abuse followed by a brief period of stability and even reconciliation, Walker offered an explanation that might be relevant to some women. However, accounts from women give the impression that in reality violence is somewhat less predictable, often occurring when least expected, and commonly not followed by attempts at reconciliation (Hester *et al.* 2000). Williamson (2000: 27) emphasizes the risk inherent in the theory of learned helplessness when applied to all women as it tends to stereotype an abused woman as one who loses her identity, suffers in silence, does not retaliate.

Key points

Women are faced with complex choices when they are making decisions about leaving violent partners. For each woman those decisions are dependent on the particular circumstances she faces (Hester *et al.* 2000: 29).

It is your responsibility as a healthcare practitioner to facilitate women to make an informed choice, not to pressure them into making a reactive, and potentially dangerous, response. Each woman must be viewed as an individual who may have developed sophisticated survival skills, which have enabled her to survive in an abusive relationship. The woman who appears assertive and vocal is probably in as much danger as the woman who is quiet and withdrawn, and their care should reflect their individual needs.

According to Mullender (1996), there is an additional predicament for women who access health and social services and then fail to act on the advice and support offered. It is a possibility that they may be deemed a less 'worthy' cause the next time they seek assistance. 'There is a common but brutal misconception that if women do not leave, the violence they are enduring cannot be all that intolerable' (Victim Support 1992: 7). Mullender describes how for many women the initial incident may not be perceived as being particularly serious, they believe that it is a one-off, or even an accident, and that it will never happen again. Over time as the incidents increase in frequency and severity, many women still have the hope that the violence will stop and many continue in the belief that one day their relationship will return to the way it was before. However, as the state of affairs continues, the realization comes that the violence has now become the norm. Some women are able to leave the violent relationship, whilst others, for a variety of reasons, may develop sophisticated coping strategies and stay.

Key point

Leaving a violent and abusive relationship is often a long and painful process and not a single desperate act, one that may carry with it the risk of dangerous, if not fatal, consequences.

The healthcare practitioner must never intervene, by word or deed, in a way that may cause the woman and/or her children further harm.

MEDIUM- AND LONG-TERM EFFECTS OF BEING ABUSED

Five per cent of health years of life are lost world-wide by women because of domestic violence.

(Social Services Inspectorate: Department of Health 1996)

A history of current or past abuse has been associated with multiple health sequelae, including injuries directly resulting from physical violence (Goldberg; Tomlanovich, 1984); increased substance use; chronic pelvic pain; abdominal/pelvic pain (Rapkin *et al.* 1990); headaches (Ratner 1995); and gastrointestinal disorders (Drossman *et al.* 1990). In addition to physical injury, Butler (1995: 55) identified that women frequently experience anxiety, fatigue, dependency, depression, sleeping and eating disorders, chronic pain and other problems as a result of living with the constant threat. Williamson (2000: 34) concurred that many women present to healthcare providers with varied psychosomatic symptoms including: sleeping disorders, neurotic behaviour, varied non-specific physical symptoms, general feelings of un-wellness and extreme fatigue.

Psychological problems

Women who are being abused often demonstrate some psychological and emotional effects in the short, medium and often long term. Often the woman experiences:

- feelings of low self-worth
- loss of self-respect
- depression
- feelings of hopelessness
- loss of confidence.

In addition:

- Some women may suffer from anxiety attacks and recurring panic attacks

- Some may even suffer from agoraphobia or claustrophobia depending upon the type of abuse they have been subjected to.
- Other women may develop self-harming behaviours.
- Research shows that a significant number of abused adults turn to drugs and alcohol as a result of the abuse.

It is generally acknowledged that abused women often continue to experience feelings of worthlessness and fear for a long time after their partner has finally left, and for some women it continues for a lifetime (Dobash and Dobash 1992, Hague and Malos 1993).

Medium- to long-term health implications for physical well-being

The immediate injuries commonly inflicted on the woman have been documented above; however, some progress to become medium- and long-term effects. Williamson (2000) acknowledged how continuous minor injuries can eventually lead to long-term problems. For example, eye injuries, including 'black eyes', are commonly sustained during an attack, but, as for a boxer, continuous injury over time can lead to permanent damage to the sight. Similarly, repeated head injuries may ultimately result in irreversible neurological deficit including stroke and partial paralysis, spinal injuries, and musculo-skeletal injury to name but a few, eventually producing long-term functional deficits.

Some women may require reconstructive surgery, especially following severe facial injuries, which of course may be so expensive as to be prohibitive, leaving the woman with the negative body image experienced by those who are disfigured. Other illnesses which may progress from immediate to medium- and long-term health deficits include: irritable bowel syndrome; sexually transmitted diseases (STDs); pelvic inflammatory disease (PID); unexplained chronic gynaecological problems, for example, vaginitis, pelvic pain, and sexual dysfunction. Women may present for healthcare with an illness which has its origins in domestic violence even though the abusive situation may have been resolved.

Domestic violence and pregnancy

Amongst a group of pregnant women attending primary care in East London: 15 per cent reported violence during their pregnancy. Just under 40 per cent reported that violence started whilst they were pregnant, whilst 30 per cent who reported violence during pregnancy also reported they had at sometime suffered a miscarriage as a result.

(Department of Health [DoH] 2000b: 41 [Dr Jeremy Coid])

Women may present with health problems either during pregnancy, or afterwards, when their recovery is compromised by the original or continuing abuse and violence. Similarly the newborn baby may suffer short-, medium- and long-term health deficits as a result of the mother being abused during pregnancy. The immediate and long-term management of pregnant women who are being abused is dealt with in more detail in Chapter 5.

Medium- to long-term health implications for emotional and psychological well-being

As we have seen above, individuals systematically abused in an intimate relationship may present with a variety of psychological and emotional health needs.

Mental health problems

Stark and Flitcraft (1996) state that women who have been abused are:

- 15 times more likely to abuse alcohol
- 5 times more likely to attempt suicide
- 9 times more likely to abuse drugs
- 3 times more likely to be diagnosed with a depressive or psychotic episode.

Substance abuse

The National Clearinghouse for Alcohol and Drug Information in advice to health professionals advises that:

> While there is no direct cause-and-effect link, the use of alcohol and other drugs by either partner is a risk factor for domestic violence. . . . [T]he Panel recommends that substance abuse treatment programs screen all clients for current and past domestic violence, including childhood physical and sexual abuse. When possible, domestic violence programs should screen clients for substance abuse.
> (See US Department of Health and Human Services, National Institute on Alcohol Abuse and Alcoholism, Eighth Special Report to the US Congress on Alcohol and Health, 1993: 245)

Post traumatic stress disorder (PTSD)

Exploring the research, Wiehe (1998: 93) concludes that many women who have suffered from domestic abuse develop PTSD in varying levels of severity.
  PTSD occurs when:

> An individual is exposed to an extreme traumatic stressor, involving direct personal experience of an event that involves actual or threatened death or serious injury, or other threats to one's physical integrity. The response of the individual to the threat involves intense fear, helplessness, or horror.

Symptoms of PTSD include:

- persistent re-experiencing of the event
- persistent avoidance of stimuli associated with the trauma
- numbing of general responsiveness
- persistent symptoms of increased arousal, e.g. acute anxiety.

(Defined by American Psychiatric Association 1994)

A more detailed discussion of the related health issues is addressed in Chapter 6.

THE FINANCIAL COST OF DOMESTIC VIOLENCE

We know that domestic violence is a prevalent and persistent social problem. It causes ill health, family breakdown, social exclusion, and death. The cost of this crime to our public services and to our communities is vast – the costs to individuals and family life is incalculable.
(Barbara Roche, Minister for Women at the Cabinet Office, 2002)

The cost of domestic violence to health and social services in the UK is estimated to be over £1 billion per year. In 1997–8, an estimated 19,910 women and 28,520 children stayed in refuges in England. A study conducted at Rush Medical Centre in Chicago in 1992 found that the average charge for medical services provided to abused women, children and older people was $1,633 per person per year. This would amount to a national annual cost of $857.3 million (Meyer 1992).

In Hackney in 1996, it was estimated that the cost of domestic violence to the local health service excluding hospitalization and medicines was £580,000 in that borough, in one year (Stanko et al. 1997). These costs did not include the additional cost to housing departments, criminal justice departments, the police, or other individuals and agencies involved in assisting abused individuals, which was estimated at over £5 million. The conservative estimates of the total breakdown costs of domestic violence against the women in the study were:

- GPs   £539,776
- Accident and Emergency attendance   £17,293
- health visitors   £26,476
- police   £540,000
- civil justice   £1,004,000
- housing   £240,000
- refuges   £410,000
- social services   £2,360,000
- health   £580,000

One needs to add to this, the cost to employers for days lost through sickness; and the ongoing financial cost if the family have to be supported outside of the family home and the overall financial costs spiral.

Areas where financial costs occur

Crisp and Stanko identified that financial costs were incurred by a range of groups including: the health services; civil justice; criminal justice; social services; housing; Women's Aid and refuge services; advice and advocacy services; friends and family; and often employers and benefits. They highlighted the need for a collective, systematic approach to collating cost data in all areas including:

- social services, including related benefits
- health services
- criminal justice services
- police services
- housing and other local government services
- voluntary services such as Women's Aid
- intervention programmes both for the abused women and children and for the male perpetrators.

Information needed to improve cost-effectiveness

The Scottish Needs Assessment Programme report on domestic violence (1997) (Davidson *et al.* 2000: 2) sets out a list of the information that would be needed to address cost-effectiveness:

- basic epidemiological data about the prevalence of domestic violence
- detection costs
- costs of training and education
- healthcare use and treatment costs
- possible averted costs as a result of better management
- possible increased costs as a result of increased detection
- costs to women themselves
- appropriate summary outcome measures by which to assess effectiveness
- changes in health-related quality of life
- information about the timing of costs and benefits so that programmes with different cost-benefit profiles can be compared.

Crisp and Stanko (2000), summarizing the findings of work on financial costing of domestic violence to date, highlighted that there is a consistent pattern in the extent of inter-partner violence. However, evaluating the cost-effectiveness of intervention programmes remains problematical, as many researchers do not include this in their study. Where data is collected there is little evidence to demonstrate that it is collated effectively.

Whilst a number of studies have identified that costs related to domestic violence are substantial, particularly to the public sector and specifically to the criminal justice system, as yet we have no definitive figures from which we can work. In addition, to date there has been little effective assessment of the costs borne either by the individual or by the multiple agencies involved, in part because national data is not always responsive enough to identify regional diversities.

> **Key point**
>
> There is an urgent need to create systems of measurement that can be used to generate baseline data against which the impact and cost-effectiveness of any intervention can be assessed . . . agencies have to be able to describe what they are doing and how they are spending existing resources.
>
> (Crisp and Stanko 2000)
>
> Healthcare providers must decide how and what data to collect in order to effectively estimate the costs of domestic violence to the service they offer. Only then are they in a position to evaluate the existing service, seek appropriate levels of funding, and plan for improvement.

IMPROVING HEALTHCARE PRACTICE: RESEARCH INTO DOMESTIC VIOLENCE AND ABUSE

The emphasis on evidence-based practice in all aspects of healthcare is recognized by all professionals as a prerequisite to effective, efficient and safe care. Therefore, in order to move forward the assessment, management and evaluation of care as it relates to domestic abuse, valid research must be placed at the top of the healthcare agenda.

A need for improvement

It should be noted that in recent years important research about many aspects of domestic violence in the United Kingdom has emerged. Nevertheless, international research studies into all aspects of domestic violence are frequently contradictory. For example, some researchers claim domestic violence is almost as common against men as it is against women. In contrast, other authors, including Mullender (1996), BMA (1999) and Women's Aid Federation (2000), to name but a few, are resolute that the problem is primarily violence against women with men as the primary perpetrators. Some of the reasons why this controversy exists are:

- There is no agreed definition of domestic violence/abuse, therefore it is often impossible or inappropriate to compare and contrast research findings.
- Many studies focus on physical violence with little reference to the other types of abuse.
- The research sample has a major impact upon the study; it may be incongruous to compare groups of abused women in the UK with those from, for example, the USA. Thus findings are often not generalizable to other groups of abused women.
- According to the BMA (1999) study, samples are often quite small and rigorous methodology is not always applied to the research, whilst the research on male perpetrators is frequently flawed.

The BMA further suggests that few tools used to measure either violence or victim responses have been adequately validated, which may compromise the validity of the data collected. For example, the Conflict Tactics Scale designed by Straus (1979) is frequently used by researchers to measure types and amounts of family violence. However, it is not without its critics; Jackson and Oates (1998: 142–3, 227), summarizing recent criticism, identify aspects of violence which are not included within the tool. For instance, the tool fails to recognize intent or purpose of violence; whether it was offensive action or defensive action; or rates of injury. Nor does it consider ethnic diversity and is thus, they claim, culturally biased. However, divergence is inevitable, for when researching a subject the research approach, the manner in which one defines and operationalizes concepts, data collection methods, sample selection and the actual research questions, all undoubtedly shape outcomes.

One of the foremost challenges of estimating the frequency of violence from an intimate partner is that it is a violation that many women will not admit to enduring. Similarly, many perpetrators never admit to being abusive. Therefore, statistics related to violence in intimate relationships are generally under-reported and thus underestimated. Professor Stanko, addressing a major criminal justice conference in 1999, highlighted that many abused women contact a wide variety of institutions and organizations, including the police, the GP, housing departments, legal aid, citizens' advice bureaux, women's organizations and other health professionals. However, because there is often little inter-agency collaboration we have no way of knowing how many women are actively seeking help at any one moment in time. Thus, current data on the size and nature of the problem is limited.

Gaps in our knowledge

According to Davidson *et al.* (2000: 2):

> There are serious limitations to our knowledge about what works in healthcare settings in decreasing the impact of domestic violence on women, and consequently what is cost-effective. There is an urgent need for evaluative research to guide us in developing policy and practice in this area.

Specifically, they identify several important gaps in our knowledge of domestic violence in the UK including:

- the extent to which domestic violence impacts on health
- the impact of intervention programmes in healthcare such as:
  - screening women to discover who is experiencing violence;
  - assessing with them their risk of serious violence;
  - what works to help them improve their lives; and what services they need;
- links between health and other services
- views of care-givers and of women
- costs of care in the health sector for victims and their families
- social and geographic variations within the UK
- the impact of violence prevention programmes.

At the time of writing, the authors found a significant paucity of research related to clinical interventions in the UK.

Key points

Many areas pertaining to domestic abuse and healthcare are under-researched in the UK. Much more needs to be known about:

- the size and nature of the phenomenon
- specific effects on the health and social welfare of diverse groups including, amongst others, black women, ethnic minority groups, men, gay, lesbian and transgender couples
- the effectiveness of specific healthcare interventions
- the efficacy of multi-agency domestic violence forums
- research related to specific clinical areas of practice such as Accident and Emergency, Obstetrics and Gynaecology, community care, GP services, mental health responses, and acute care management
- the causes of intimate violence and the effectiveness of intervention programmes.

In addition, the BMA recommend that a central data base of domestic violence research and projects should be established for access by researchers, professional healthcare personnel, academics and agencies dealing with domestic violence. The current government (2003) has taken important steps in the work of informing healthcare staff, encouraging multi-agency collaboration, and supporting the police services in their endeavours related to domestic abuse, but a greater part remains unaccomplished.

Chapter 3

Abuse in other intimate relationships

Current UK statistics relating to domestic violence within intimate relationships other than between a heterosexual couple are somewhat limited, as is the research. However, whilst it is widely accepted that violence between intimate partners is predominantly male against female, there is increasing acknowledgement that domestic violence is on occasions perpetrated by women against men, and occurs within same-sex relations. Equally, there is a range of clients who, because of their individual circumstances, possess explicit needs. This chapter explores domestic violence and abuse in the context of women's abuse against men, and abuse in same-sex and transgender relationships. It will also investigate the specific challenges related to domestic abuse faced by women of colour, and other women whose ethnicity determines the patriarchal structure of family, marriage, and partnerships. Finally, the chapter focuses on the manner in which religious tenets can influence family structures and thus the responses of individuals within an abusive relationship.

FEMALE VIOLENCE AND ABUSE AGAINST MEN

According to the Mirlees-Black British Crime Survey (BCS) (1999), 14.9 per cent of men surveyed reported being victims of domestic violence, compared to 22.7 per cent of the women surveyed. In *Criminal Statistics for England and Wales* (1997), it was noted that 8 per cent of male homicide victims were killed by their female partners, in contrast to 47 per cent of women killed by their male partners or ex-partners.

Key point

To deny that women can, and do on occasions, subject their male partners to violence and abuse would be naive in the extreme. There can be no doubt that some women can, and do, bully and intimidate their male partners to the point where the man requires outside intervention. The man may have to resort to accessing legal services, including the police service, and to health services. Nevertheless, there can be no doubt that the vast majority of violence within intimate relationships is perpetrated by men against women.

However, studies generally agree that female-on-male violence and male-on-female violence differ significantly in type, frequency, duration, and the degree of physical damage inflicted. Even less is known about the existence of, or nature of, any psychological, emotional or sexual abuse that women may inflict upon men.

In the 1999 BCS survey of men and women between the ages of 16 and 59, Walby and Myhill (2000: 1) noted that women were significantly more affected than men in the following areas:

- twice as often injured in the attack
- more often subjected to frightening threats
- more prone to severe physical injury and to multiple attacks
- upset and frightened by the attack.

These findings were supported by Mullender (1996: 13). Moreover, other studies have established that women also endure sexual assault and rape, are frequently subjected to prolonged emotional abuse, and are far more apt to be mortally wounded.

When women are violent towards men, much of the existing research indicates that their violence is often a defence against violence towards them. Alternatively, as we have seen in cases widely noted by the press, women may kill their partner after years of severe mental, physical and sexual violence, when they fear for their lives. Women's violence may be defensive, but when men hit women, the assault is often potentially life-threatening (Mullender 1996: 15).

Statistics related to domestic violence towards men remain inconclusive and, on occasions, quite contradictory. A high proportion of the data has emerged from the USA, including the first national Survey on Family Violence in 1975, and more recently the MORI poll undertaken in the UK by the *Here and Now* television programme. Both studies utilized the Conflict Tactics Scale (CRS) research instrument and concluded that women and men were equally prone to using violence against their partner. However, the studies have been severely criticized and challenged by the academic community for lack of validity and reliability. Sexual assault was not included on the scale, many of the themes were not clearly defined, and the results were open to wide interpretation.

As the BMA (1999: 26) indicates, a slap from a muscular man has the potential to cause far greater physical injury than a slap from a female, demonstrating that a particular act can have quite varied consequences. Critics further argue that to ignore the social context of domestic violence does little to augment the debate or improve services for those in need of protection.

Key point

What is essential for all healthcare practitioners to take into account is that whilst the debate about definitions, severity, and causes continues there are men accessing health services today who are being abused by their female partner. Therefore, when designing local protocols, staff development programmes, or advice sheets for clients, staff must take into account abuse against men if the service is to be equitable and meaningful across all user groups.

VIOLENCE IN GAY, LESBIAN, BISEXUAL AND TRANSGENDER RELATIONSHIPS

Whilst it is generally acknowledged that domestic violence exists in gay, lesbian, bisexual and transgender relationships (GLBT), rather less is known about the specific problems this may cause for the abused individual. As yet, there is also little known about the patterns of violence, the contributory factors, or the dynamics of violence within such relationships. Clients within a GLBT relationship, abused by their partner or ex-partner, have the added burden of existing in a society that continues to be judgemental and often condemnatory of such relationships. For example, in law, gay and lesbian couples have even fewer rights than do men and women within an abusive heterosexual relationship, and may also be faced with hostility and prejudice when seeking help. In the United States, Jackson and Oates (1998) identify nine states that have domestic violence laws which still apply only to heterosexual couples.

Moreover, if it is not widely known that the abused partner is gay, she or he may have to live under the threat of being 'outed', as part of the control and abuse. Jackson and Oates (1998) define this type of abuse as heterosexist control. In a world that remains in many spheres homophobic, it is unsurprising that gay men and women may prefer to keep their sexual orientation unknown.

Key point

If the healthcare practitioner suspects that a client is being abused, she or he should try to ensure that the client is left alone with the doctor or nurse, if only for a short while. However, practitioners unaware of the complexity of abusive relationships may not be concerned about the 'friend' who stays close by to offer comfort and support. Imagine, however, if this loyal friend is in fact the abusive partner. If one assumes domestic violence only happens to heterosexual women, then many other individuals are left isolated and at risk of harm.

Male-to-male violence

Research suggests that between 25 and 30 per cent of all gay men and lesbian women in intimate relationships suffer abuse at some point in their relationship (Letellier 1994: 16), a similiar ratio to that which occurs in heterosexual partnerships. Burke (1998), summarizing the research on intimate violence amongst gay couples, concluded that:

- Domestic violence in gay partnerships is a serious health concern.
- Within the gay community, domestic violence is a major health need second only to acquired immune deficiency disease and substance abuse.
- In a study of 1,000 gay men 17 per cent had experienced some form of abuse from their partner (Elliott 1996).
- In the USA, out of approximately 12 million gay adult males, 500,000 are thought to suffer violence from their partner.
- More gay men are killed by their partner than by a stranger (Letellier 1994: 95).

- The causes of intimate violence in gay male relationships are thought to be very similar to those in lesbian and in heterosexual relationships.
- The law related to domestic violence often excludes abuse within gay male relationships or lesbian relationships.
- Vandalism – the threat of, or act of, destroying property especially that which has great sentimental value – is not uncommon in gay relationships.
- Violence may extend, as it does in other abusive intimate relationships, to harming pets as a means of exerting power and control.
- As death from AIDS is more common in male homosexuals, according to L. Smith (1989) an infected abused man may remain in the relationship for fear of dying alone, given his dependence on the abuser.
- Similarly, the man being abused may feel unable to leave his partner if the partner is HIV positive or has AIDS.
- Where the abusive partner is infected with the HIV virus, physically or emotionally forcing the partner to have unprotected sex is arguably the ultimate in control.

Violence within lesbian relationships

The 'myth that women are not violent,' is persistent and contributes to a denial of woman-to-woman sexual violence, not only among the general population but also among lesbians. 'We want to believe that our relationships are safe, that we have equality, and that we have ideal communities. But it's not true.'
(Professor Girshwick. Professor of Sociology and Women's Studies at Warren Wilson College in North Carolina, November 2000)

Whilst the feminist movement was the inspirational force in establishing domestic violence on the international agenda, according to Jackson and Oates (1998), the same faction has been slow to acknowledge the plight of lesbian women within abusive relationships. Lesbian women who are living in, or have recently exited, an abusive relationship may have experienced many of the abusive behaviours identified above. Additional issues for lesbian women could include:

- a general disquiet from the lesbian community about making public violence in lesbian partnerships
- suffering sexual abuse at the hands of their female partner
- being threatened with the loss of their children
- not getting support from their lesbian friends, as many would prefer to keep the whole issues of lesbian abuse quiet
- being not necessarily safe in a refuge; whilst men are excluded totally, an abusive woman may possibly be persuasive and gain entry
- as there are few refuges which cater solely for lesbian women, they may have the added burden of seeking refuge only to be met with homophobic hostility
- receiving legal assistance may not be easy, as most police initiatives have focused on male violence against women.

DOMESTIC VIOLENCE AND WOMEN WITH DISABILITIES

> A recent national study by the Center for Research on Women with Disabilities shows that women with physical disabilities experience about the same rate of emotional, physical, and sexual abuse as women without disabilities.
>
> (Young *et al.* 1997: 78)

This and other studies show that women with disabilities who are being abused also tend to have an additional set of challenges because of their disability.

Summarizing, the study showed that:

- A greater number of women with disabilities experience the abuse over longer periods than do non-disabled women.
- The most common perpetrators are husbands, male partners, or live-in companions.
- Women with disabilities more frequently experience abuse by medical professionals, and by parents, than women without disabilities.
- Abuse has a more severe negative effect on the self-esteem of women with physical disabilities than those without disabilities.
- There are those, often including the disabled person, who believe it is the pressure of caring that causes the abuser to lose their temper. This of course is vigorously challenged by theorists.

Furthermore, Mullender (1996) indicates that the woman may continue to tolerate the abuse for fear of losing her children, as alone she may be unable to care for them. The way in which the women in the study said that they were abused was also significant, a number reporting a new dimension of abuse, called *disability-related abuse*, in which perpetrators withhold essential support including:

- equipment such as wheelchairs, or braces
- medications
- transportation, so that the woman is kept virtually a hostage in the home
- essential assistance with personal tasks, such as dressing or getting out of bed.

Depending upon the severity of disability the perpetrator of the abuse may be in a position of almost absolute power. The woman may be totally dependent upon her carer for support in maintaining her daily living activities, for her social activities and her emotional and psychological well-being. The carer may perhaps be in a position to intervene between the healthcare provider and the client, ensuring the abuse is kept hidden. Moreover, the woman is often financially dependent upon the abuser and seeking appropriate refuge is therefore even more challenging. People with severe physical disabilities are frequently limited in their social interactions, and the woman may have endured the abuse for so long she believes it to be a normal part of her life.

Financial dependence due to disability

Disabled people are more likely to be in low paid jobs or living on low incomes. Disabled people make up 12 per cent of all people in employment. However, disabled people are half as likely as non-disabled people to be in paid work.

> (Greater London Action on Disability [GLAD] 1995: 2)

Women with learning disabilities are, according to the BMA (1998), particularly vulnerable to domestic abuse especially sexual abuse as they often have poor levels of sex education. According to the BMA (1999), there is little recognition amongst professional groups, including disability groups, of the issues related to intimate violence and abuse amongst this frequently vulnerable group. Insufficient knowledge or influence to bring about change means that the status quo has existed unchecked for a long time.

HEALTHCARE INTERVENTION

> The oppression of disabled women and the exploitation of women carers are compounded if specialist workers in every field of disability do not know how to recognize and respond with appropriate urgency and sensitivity to domestic abuse or do not look for it.
>
> (Mullender 1996: 134)

Studies indicate that besides the usual reasons for not intervening, health and social care staff often consider the abuse to be a family matter believing the victim will ask for help if she needs it. This may be particularly true if the couple have been together for many years. All too often if abuse appears to be long-standing, 'outsiders' naively assume that it cannot be that bad, otherwise the woman would leave. Moreover, the woman quite probably believes that if the choice is staying where she is, or going into a home, staying is the 'lesser of two evils'. She may also feel intimidated by the reports of institutional abuse she may have read in the press or seen on television.

In contrast, Mullender (1996) also points out that the person with the disability may be male and abusing his female partner, but as the carer, she feels far too guilty to walk out and leave him to fend for himself. Equally, the same scenario might occur if the abuser who is disabled is female, and the carer male, or if they are a homosexual or gay couple. Mullender further supports the view that women with learning difficulties are especially vulnerable to sexual abuse. Moreover, arrest and prosecution of the offender is extremely difficult, and in many cases prohibitive, as the woman may be viewed as a non-credible witness.

Key point

Where health practitioners become aware, or suspect, that a client with a disability is suffering abuse from their partner, working with other professionals such as social services and housing benefits officers is essential if the intervention is to be successful. Perhaps more importantly, any attempts by the professionals to intercede must take place with the full consent and co-operation of the disabled person. All too often individuals and groups with disabilities are left feeling totally powerless in the face of 'professional intervention'.

Nosek (1999) devised a set of guidelines for healthcare practitioners to recognize and deal with the needs of clients with disabilities who are currently suffering, or have in the past suffered, abuse at the hands of a partner. These guidelines are based on the work of Salber and Taliaferro (1995). The guide suggests that the reasons why the women do not ask for help are very similar to those of non-disabled women; however, in addition the woman fears the consequences of disclosure.

Often an individual with a disability is dependent upon her or his partner, who may also act as carer. She or he may fear being left alone and that no one in the future will want a relationship with her or him. Imagine how it might be for the disabled person unable to leave the house without assistance, with no escape from the relentless name-calling, the psychological battering, the constant ridicule and threats. It is not difficult to see why a woman in this situation could, after a relatively short period, become convinced that there is no way out and therefore adopt sophisticated strategies for survival, including that of denial.

Where the healthcare practitioner is alerted to such a scenario, it is imperative that he or she takes advice from members of the multi-disciplinary team before intervening. To make it known to the perpetrator that their actions have been noted could severely compromise the health and safety of the client. Where possible the health worker needs to arrange a meeting alone with the woman. However, how, when and where this takes place should be carefully planned. Literature related to abuse should only be left with the client if she or he is confident that they can either explain its presence or keep it in a place where it cannot be found by the partner. Arguably, if domestic violence literature were given out to all users of the health service on a regular basis the perpetrator would in all probability take less notice. Where women's groups, mother and toddler groups, support, and activity groups for the elderly, or the disabled, and groups for young people meet, the literature should be made easily accessible. In fact, domestic violence information must be available wherever it is usual to have health promotion literature displayed, in public places such as the library, surgeries, council offices and benefit offices.

Key point

Mullender (1996) draws attention to the fact that information delivered in traditional written form on posters and leaflets or in verbal form via television adverts does not meet the needs of all client groups. Whilst many organizations offer materials in a variety of languages few present it in a form that is useful for clients with hearing or sight impairments.

It is important to recognize the limitations of written information given to those with poor sight or blindness who might need it in large print, Braille or on tape. Equally a deaf woman may require the services of someone who can sign with or for her, if her needs are to be adequately assessed and appropriate interventions planned with her.

CURRENT PRACTICE

The following extract from GLAD (Greater London Action on Disability 1995) sums up some of the numerous difficulties faced by a disabled individual attempting to flee an abusive home life. Whilst these statistics relate specifically to London there is no evidence that disabled people elsewhere in the UK fare any better.

> Very few of London's refuges offer accessible accommodation or adaptations for women with sensory impairments. Those refuges that are accessible (and the one refuge that provides for women with learning difficulties) are under considerable pressure. There are no reciprocal arrangements between boroughs for transferring care packages if a woman has to flee a violent situation. Nor do Police domestic violence specialist units receive any Disability Equality Training.

Information available from GLAD, and other organizations fighting for the rights of people with disabilities, highlights the chronic lack of facilities of any kind for disabled people without adding the burden of an abusive home life. It is therefore understandable if women with disabilities find the thought of leaving an abusive home even more threatening than staying.

Mullender (1996) criticizes past approaches to care for abused disabled people for whom the supporting organizations offered respite care or additional support as a solution to the violence. This type of intervention presupposes that the violence and abuse have been precipitated by the stress of caring for the dependent person, as opposed to defining it as a criminal act. This approach might possibly be useful in the short term as it gives the disabled person a respite from the violence but it does nothing to change the perpetrator.

Other research has criticized the lack of facilities in refuges for disabled women; some do not even have wheelchair access. Refuges are rarely purpose built, and they are established and maintained on a limited budget, refuge priorities being quite low on the local authority agenda. To equip refuges for easy access would be cost prohibitive in many areas, further discriminating against abused women with disabilities.

Key point

Healthcare organisations must ensure staff at all levels are aware of the particular challenges for individuals with disabilities who are in abusive relationships. Staff must recognize that this client group is at even greater risk if their disability is such that it makes it impossible to leave the house if the violence escalates. Policies and procedures which acknowledge both the client need and the preferred multi-agency interventions must be in place.

DOMESTIC VIOLENCE AGAINST WOMEN FROM BLACK AND MINORITY ETHNIC GROUPS IN THE UNITED KINGDOM

There is a lack of understanding of the cultural needs of black and minority ethnic women experiencing domestic violence, including language difficulties and financial dependence on husbands. Many such women are unaware of refuges. They may fear racism in mixed refuges, but this fear is lessened if there are black and minority ethnic staff.

(Sally Keeble, Housing Minister, May 2002)

Since the 1970s, when domestic violence was first acknowledged in the UK as a social phenomenon, significant research studies have been undertaken. Whilst theorists and practitioners may continue to debate the possible definitions, causes, preconditions, levels and types of intervention or the societal sub-groups who are abused, it is generally acknowledged that women from different cultures, ethnic groups and/or religions have specific needs. But, despite popular myths, no one group of women is any more prone to abuse than another and whilst there may exist elements on which we are able to generalize, it must be acknowledged that each woman has quite specific individual needs. Moreover, it is important to note that according to Mama (2000: 48): All manner of non-white households are causally depicted as black families: families from India, Guyana, Jamaica, St Kitts, Ghana, Uganda, Morocco, Somalia, and other countries live in a post-colonial Britain which views them as black. However, Mama emphasizes that not all black women, and not all Asian women, share the same religious and cultural norms and beliefs, in the same way neither do all white women. Therefore, where assumptions, policies and practices related to domestic violence are based on skin colour or racial stereotypes, they are inevitably discriminatory and harmful to the women they are supposed to help. This section aims, where possible and when possible, to address the needs of as many diverse groups as it can.

Throughout Britain, dedicated help lines and women's refuges are being established for women from black and minority ethnic groups. Among them are the Southall Black Women group, and groups for Asian women, Jewish women, Chinese women, Turkish women. However, such facilities are few and far between, and many women in violent relationships do not have sufficient local support. More recently, groups with specialist knowledge to aid women seeking asylum, refugee women and women from other countries who have married British men, have been established and are seeking to meet the needs of these groups of women. Similarly, work is being undertaken to distinguish the needs of older women and disabled women, again appreciating that they have specific physical, psychological and social needs.

As a multicultural society, people in Britain must understand that an abused woman can be from any age group, any social stratum, any race, any culture and, indeed, any lifestyle. What is apparent from reading the literature is the different manner in which women from different black and minority ethnic groups define and/or respond to domestic violence. In a study undertaken in a North London borough by Mooney in 1993, it was confirmed that domestic violence cuts across race and ethnicity. However, the study highlighted distinctions both in definition, and in patterns of reporting, across different ethnic groups. For example, African Caribbean women regularly defined all the behaviours cited in the researcher's definition as domestic violence:

- 97 per cent agreed that it included mental cruelty
- 85 per cent agreed that it included being made to have sex without giving consent
- 90 per cent included physical violence that did not result in actual bodily harm
- 52 per cent had reported incidents to a formal agency.

The latter finding was in contrast to Mama's study (2000), which concluded that

> black women may be particularly reluctant to seek outside help: many endure a high level of abuse over long periods rather than run the risk of homelessness and its attendant vulnerability, hardship and indignity, not to mention the bureaucratic intransigence.
>
> (Mama 2000: 48)

whereas, English, Scottish and Welsh women had the third lowest reporting rate to agencies and, generally, they did not report the abuse to friends or relatives. Furthermore, no African women had reported abusive incidents to the police, only 67 per cent of African women would include mental cruelty, and only 55 per cent would include 'being made to have sex without consent' in their definition of domestic violence. Similarly, the study identified that Irish women tended not to categorize rape as domestic violence. Women in the other categories, i.e. African, Turkish, Asian, Greek, and Cypriot, were averse to including this as domestic violence and were the least likely group to report to either agencies or friends/relatives. This study was carried out in the UK. Findings in the United States proffer quite different statistics and to gain a wider perspective one would need to read more widely about domestic violence in other countries.

Key point

To understand the wider needs of clients in abusive relationships, the healthcare practitioner should take the time to read literature on providing appropriate healthcare which meets the specific needs of persons from diverse ethnic, cultural and religious groups. This is of particular relevance when dealing with women in abusive and violent relationships, when ignorance of their needs could lead to misunderstandings.

How we define and thus research into the subject of domestic violence, in particular across international and ethnic boundaries, offers a significant challenge to quantifying the type, frequency, severity and consequence of violence against women generally, and especially in specific groups. Undertaking comparative analysis of existing data is fraught with difficulty and without including the social context of each group or country, it is perhaps an exercise of limited value.

Oates (1998: 226) illustrates how people from ethnic minority groups having their own culture, traditions, values and beliefs, which may be quite different from the majority group, may frequently experience negative attitudes and ideas from that majority. Oates further argues that past research on violence in families undertaken in the USA was underpinned by cultural bias that promulgated a belief that violence occurs more frequently and with greater severity in minority families, specifically African American families. Mama (2000) supports this premise in her critique of research studies with erroneous portrayals of stereotypical black families, white families or families of mixed race.

SPECIFIC HEALTHCARE NEEDS OF WOMEN FROM BLACK AND MINORITY ETHNIC GROUPS

Whenever women from black and minority ethnic groups access healthcare facilities with conditions related to domestic violence, it is probable that they have specific needs. Their individual needs may depend upon whether or not they were born in the United Kingdom:

- Some women do not have English as a first language. Therefore, this may be a barrier when seeking and receiving services. Where possible interpreters should be found, but asking a member of the family, or a friend, to interpret may act as a barrier. The woman may be either unable or too afraid to discuss her situation openly and honestly.
- Whilst the woman's community or religion probably does not actually support violence or abuse, nevertheless, members of that community may apply pressure on the woman to either stay in the marriage, or stay quiet. Religious and community leaders in all cultures tend to be men and only some speak out against violence.
- Women from some minority ethnic groups may feel they have too much to lose by leaving. For instance, religious or cultural beliefs may forbid divorce, considering separation and divorce to be a family disgrace.
- Black women and women from minority ethnic communities may be wary of involving the police/legal system or other services because of racism within institutions which is manifested in a variety of ways. Many of these women may have already suffered first-hand from social and institutional racism.
- The cultural setting in which domestic violence occurs affects the way the woman experiences it. Sensitivity to any differences is important; understanding and respecting the views and wishes of the woman must be of paramount concern.
- Moving to a refuge is a traumatic experience for any woman. Imagine how it must feel to the woman who cannot speak the language, or whose way of life is totally different to that of others in the home.
- There are a few specialist refuges for black and minority ethnic women. All refuges should confront the issue of racism, but some women may not feel supported, or may experience blatant racism or cultural misunderstandings in refuges. However, there may be women who would prefer to go to a mixed refuge, therefore one should not make assumptions about individual preference.
- Black and minority ethnic women might be able to find people in their community to support them. In locations where there exists a large ethnic community, there may be a women's group for women from that community. For example, in Coventry where there is a large Asian community, a specialist refuge exists. Equally the woman seeking help should be advised to consider carefully to whom she divulges her whereabouts if she is forced to seek refuge. The woman she shares the information with may feel compelled to reveal the secret to her family, depending on where the individual's loyalties lie.
- Some women from black and minority ethnic groups may never have had to deal with local authorities, banks or building societies and may feel overwhelmed at the prospect.

(Adapted from the web pages of Greenwich County Council, London Borough of Greenwich (2002))

POTENTIAL DIFFICULTIES FACED BY WOMEN FROM AN ASIAN CULTURE

In recent years we have read in the national press many stories of how young Asian women have been forced into 'arranged marriages', some even being made to go abroad to marry a man chosen by their family. Historically, in this and other countries there has often been a general reluctance on the part of legal, social, political and health services to intervene in what was deemed a matter for the specific religious and cultural community. For many Asian women their esteem from self and others is based upon their marital status. To separate from one's lawful husband is to bring disgrace to the family:

> For Asian women the decision is especially hard. The stigma of being divorced or separated has very grave consequences, as a woman's respectability, status and honour is dependent on her marital status. Notions of honour (*izzat*) and shame (*sharam*) play an important role in containing and policing many Asian women. Honour means reputation, respectability, and status. Women are considered the upholders of the honour of the family and it is their behaviour which becomes the mark of family honour.
> (http://www.ncadc.org.uk/letters/news8/domvio.html Greater Manchester Legal Aid)

Women in this situation may often find themselves completely isolated, cut off from friends and family and without funds to support themselves. Women from other religious backgrounds may find themselves in similar isolating situations, as the tenets of many religions support the 'honourable' status of marriage and actively discourage separation and divorce.

Key point

Successful healthcare intervention depends on the healthcare provider having empathy and understanding of the client's individual circumstances. Therefore, health providers must ensure that their provision meets the needs of all of the local community. This can be achieved by providing services that are culturally sensitive, in a language easily accessible to the local ethnic groups.

SPECIFIC ISSUES FOR MIGRANT WOMEN

> Some black and ethnic minority women may be particularly inhibited from reporting domestic violence because of the provisions of immigration legislation . . . the woman is likely to be fearful of using either the criminal or civil justice system because she realises that she is at risk of being required to leave the country, and believes that the authorities will take action against her.
> (Mike O'Brien, The Parliamentary Under-Secretary of State for the Home Department, *23 Jul 1999: Column: 680*, Members in the Commons, Hansard Written Answers)

It is essential that not all women from black or minority ethnic groups are perceived as recent migrants. Similarly, neither should it be assumed that all migrant women are black; to do so leads to some women with specific needs being offered inappropriate guidance and help. Immigration law is extremely complex and therefore if the client who is being abused is a recent immigrant, who either does not yet have a legal right to remain in Britain or is unsure of their current status, professional legal advice should be sought without delay.

The one-year rule

When an individual enters the UK to join their spouse who is either a British citizen or has right of residence in the UK, the Home Office gives the marriage a one-year trial period. Such is the case even if the couple have already been married for a period of time, but not lived in the UK, and this is often referred to as the *one-year rule*. After a year in the UK, the spouse who either is a British citizen or has right of residence in the UK can apply for their spouse to have the legal right to settle in the UK. However, if the marriage ends within the year, the non-settled spouse loses her entitlement to settle in the UK. This was originally implemented to ensure that 'marriages of convenience' entered into in order that one party might claim the right to residency in the UK, did not take place. If the position is reversed and it is the male partner seeking to stay, he may put extreme pressure on the woman to remain within an abusive marriage whilst he awaits his permanent residence status.

Because of these anomalies, certain women's groups have applied pressure to government ministers; in 1999 the government made a 'concessionary policy' which in effect states that in certain circumstances the one-year rule may be waived. Women who can prove that they have been abused (usually physically) by their husband during this one-year period and have either had to leave, or have been excluded from, the marital home by their husband, may appeal against deportation. This may be an intensely difficult, if not impossible, task for the abused woman with no easy access to legal assistance. Often the woman does not speak the language and may be totally unaware that violence against a spouse is illegal in this country. Moreover, even after the one year has expired and the couple are still together, the husband does not have to apply immediately to the Home Office for permanent residency for his wife. This can occasionally be used as a threat by the male partner to maintain control over the wife.

Individuals seeking to stay in the United Kingdom may have limited, rights of access to health and social care provision. They may be excluded from accessing, primary healthcare, and housing benefit making it exceedingly difficult for a woman to leave the marital home. Added to the burden of possibly not being able to speak the language, lack of access to her passport and other legal documents, having no outside contacts and often being financially totally dependent upon the husband for money, the woman may have no alternative but to stay in an abusive environment.

REFUGEES AND ASYLUM SEEKERS

The legislation as it refers to the rights of those seeking asylum or refugee status in the UK is extremely complex, changeable and, in recent years, controversial. Because of continuing international disequilibrium, many people have left their own country and seek a new life in another more stable and often more prosperous one. One of the many challenges for the immigration authorities is the need to determine between those individuals who are seeking refuge because they are in fear of their lives and those who are seeking refuge on economic grounds. This group of displaced persons may have limited or no access to benefits, healthcare and social care and may be reluctant in the extreme to access the legal system, including the police service. For illegal immigrants the plight is even more challenging, as they have no recourse to justice without the fear of deportation and permanent exclusion from the United Kingdom. Specialist advice in this situation is available from the Joint Council for the Welfare of Immigrants.

Key point

In order to offer appropriate and non-judgemental care and advice to abused clients, healthcare personnel must acknowledge and attempt to grasp the significance of ethnic, cultural and religious diversity in the assessment and intervention process.

POSSIBLE INFLUENCES OF RELIGION AND CULTURE ON DOMESTIC VIOLENCE AND ABUSE

Religion can serve as a potential roadblock or a resource in addressing issues of domestic violence. . . . [T]here are teachings which if misused and distorted, may suggest that domestic violence may be acceptable or even God's will. When these interpretations of scripture are misused they become a roadblock to ending the abuse.
(Centre for Prevention of Sexual and Domestic Violence [CPSDV] October 1994
www.cpsdv.org)

As we have seen earlier, many women, particularly once married, adopt a role subservient to that of men. They undertake most, if not all, of the domestic tasks including responsibility for raising the children, supporting elderly relatives and supporting the husband in all of his endeavours. Where this role is accepted or even expected and endorsed by her religious faith, it is predictable that the woman may receive little if any support should she decide to leave a violent and abusive partner.

Many faith-based groups and organizations have strong relationships with communities of colour, older women, women with disabilities and immigrant communities and are often supportive. Nevertheless, there are circumstances when their influence is so powerful it may cause conflict with victim advocates (Yoshioka and Dang 2000).

Religious beliefs in some relationships may play a significant role in how men and women perceive their roles within marriage or relationships, particularly in matters of power and control. Giblin (1999: 14), notes how the Catholic Church continues to: 'Emphasise church teaching of the ideal marriage, failing to acknowledge the underside of the teaching and its presumptions about sex roles, especially about dominance and submission.' Giblin goes on to say that: 'Church leaders on the national and Roman levels do not discuss the institutionalised ways in which church teaching may perpetuate sexism and contribute (even if unintentionally) to the ideological justification of violence against women.'

Whilst Giblin focuses on the role of the Roman Catholic Church, writers from other religious groups offer similar criticisms on other faith systems. For example:

> Jewish women do not come forward, in part, because it is not clear that the community will support them. The premise that a Jewish husband would never harm his wife or children has been so widely accepted that reports of abuse by Jewish men are usually met with disbelief.
>
> (Jewish Women International 1996)

Many Jewish women feel a heavy responsibility for *shalom bayit* – peace in the home – and should they fail to achieve this feel they have brought a *shanda* (shame) to the home. According to the Jewish Women Organization in the United States, studies have estimated that 15 to 20 per cent of Jewish women are abused, a rate comparable to that for non-Jewish women. The few studies that have been undertaken appear to suggest that there is no denominational difference, i.e. that the rate of violence is the same, between Orthodox, Conservative, and Reform Jews (http://www.jewishwomen.org).

For those of the Jewish faith, as in other faiths, their religious beliefs structure their entire approach to life and relationships. For example, celebrating religious holidays is seen to be an essential part of family and temple life; however, for women who have had to flee their homes and seek refuge, celebrating with friends and families is no longer an option and sadly this may be interpreted by some as desertion of the community. For many families with strong religious ties, their life is structured around the community, which shares their faith, so the woman who has to leave her home may also be surrendering her family and friends. Moreover, for the Jewish woman, the control does not cease if she leaves the marital home:

> In fact, it often escalates. Jewish divorce or *get*, as it has been interpreted over the centuries by male rabbis, can provide abusive men with yet another form of control. By refusing to grant a Jewish divorce, the man renders his wife an *agunah*, who according to Jewish law may not remarry. He, however, can do so.
>
> (Antonelli and Pearl 1996: 2)

Radford and Cappel (2001), in their study of domestic violence within the Methodist community in the UK, found that more than one in six Methodist members have personally experienced domestic violence. According to the findings of the study, many saw a conflict in the Church's thinking on marriage, endurance, redemption, forgiveness and violence. All the survivors interviewed said they stayed longer with abusive partners because they felt they had an extra responsibility to preserve their marriages.

What may be common to many religious communities was that: 'Christian forgiveness was mostly seen to mean continuing to welcome an abuser as a member of the Church while an ex-partner was excluded from Church attendance by fear' (Radford and Cappel 2001: 2). Commenting on the findings, church leaders expressed the hope that in the near future domestic violence, including training for the denomination's clergy, would be high on the agenda.

The Jehovah's Witness publication *Watchtower* states quite clearly that violence of any sort, and against one's wife specifically, is condemned, although it does imply that should a woman leave her spouse she should remain unmarried:

> Should the battered wife leave her husband? The Bible does not treat marital separation lightly. At the same time, it does not oblige a battered wife to stay with a man who jeopardises her health and perhaps her very life. The Christian apostle Paul wrote: '*If she should actually depart,* let her remain unmarried or else make up again with her husband.' (1 Corinthians 7: 10–16) Since the Bible does not forbid separation in extreme circumstances, what a woman does in this matter is a personal decision (Galatians 6: 5). No one should coax a wife to leave her husband, but neither should anyone pressure a battered woman to stay with an abusive man when her health, life, and spirituality are threatened.
>
> (*Watchtower* November 2001)

CHINESE COMMUNITIES

In a major study in the United States, Yoshioka and Dang (2000) found that in the respondents from the Chinese communities (in the USA), group participants said that many 'believe in fate and destiny', and that this orientation may contribute to an acceptance of difficult family situations. Chinese families are paternalistic and value social status, community reputation and respect for the aged. Consequently, respondents felt that Chinese families tend to 'keep bad things in the closet'. In addition, in many Chinese communities, there is strong social pressure on women to stay with their children and family and not to get divorced, as the community as a whole believes that divorce brings shame on the family name. Similar pressures are applied to women from other religious or cultural groups. Another reason given for women staying in a violent marriage was that they might be afraid of growing old and being single.

The study went on to identify how members of a Korean focus group pointed out that Buddhism and Confucianism are important in Korean culture. Such religious teachings emphasize the 'cycle of life' in which men are the rulers of the family, receiving more privilege. Moreover, 'accepting one's lot' is fundamental to their belief system and hardship is often viewed as a pathway to 'heaven', thus convincing the women that the violence is acceptable. Similarly, the study highlighted how the beliefs of Cambodian and Vietnamese women, raised to accept the dominant role of their male partners, impacted on their views of what was 'normal' behaviour within a marriage.

Yick and Agbayai-Siewert's study in 1997, involving a number of Asian communities in the USA, a survey of 31 Chinese families by telephone, demonstrated that whilst the respondents disapproved of violence overall, about 50 per cent felt that violence was justified in certain situations. These included learning of a wife's extramarital affair, a wife's losing emotional control, or gender role violations such as a wife's making a financial decision without her husband's approval. Perhaps not surprisingly, older respondents and men were more tolerant of the use of force as a means of resolving family conflict.

Equally, in a Korean community in the United States, Rhee (1997) discovered prominent Korean cultural factors and family values that may influence the development of attitudes supportive of family violence. As in other Asian communities, historically roles

GLENFIELD
MEDICAL LIBRARY

within the family were extremely patriarchal; however, Rhee noted that as many more women from these families join the labour market this is causing disequilibrium.

THE MUSLIM RELIGION

> Islam's mandate of equality between women and men necessitates that all forms of violence against women be eradicated, for so long as women suffer abuses, women cannot achieve their full potential as free and equal members of society.
>
> (Muslim Women's League, Los Angeles, March 1995)

Nevertheless, violence within a Muslim partnership is thought to occur with similar frequency to that of other religions and cultures.

> Based on information from Muslim leaders, social workers, and activists in North America, the North American Council for Muslim Women says that approximately 10 per cent of Muslim women are abused emotionally, physically, and sexually by their Muslim husbands. (There are no hard numbers, because community leaders haven't taken the well-known problem seriously enough to research.)
>
> (K. Memon, Belfast Islamic Centre)

Reading various religious texts it seems apparent that one could interpret certain passages of a number of 'Holy Books' to mean that the male has the power to chastise his wife if she fails to fulfil her wifely duties. For example, men who follow the Christian faith could find passages in the Bible which appear to support male domination and even condone violence against a woman. As in many doctrines, what is acknowledged as the 'written word' is often open to interpretation, so fundamentalists may choose to follow the letter rather than the spirit of the 'holy' word.

FORCED MARRIAGES

What is undoubtedly a small, but nevertheless significant, problem in the UK is the number of young people who are being forced into arranged marriages. Some young Muslim men and women are even being forced to go abroad to their family's country of origin, to marry and sometimes never return. When a young Muslim girl in Glasgow sought an annulment of such a marriage, the judge stated that:

> It may be that in the multi-cultural society in which we now live such situations will continue to arise where ancient Eastern established cultural and religious ethics clash with the spirit of 21st century children of a new generation and Western ideas, language and what these days passes for culture.
>
> (Judge Lord McEwan, BBC on-line, April 2002)

For many years, the courts across the UK were reluctant to intervene in matters that were defined as 'cultural and religious issues'. More recently the Labour government has called for increased vigilance from the authorities in protecting young women and men from forced marriages:

> Police forces throughout England and Wales have been ordered to treat forced marriages as a 'significant issue' under new guidelines which recommend direct intervention. Drawn up by ministers and the Association of Chief Police Officers, the guidelines state that forced marriages should be recognized as a serious abuse. Senior officers admitted they had made mistakes in the past by being 'over sensitive' to the views of elders in the ethnic community, rather than seeing the issue as a violation of human rights.
> (Sarah Womack, Social Affairs Correspondent, *Daily Telegraph*, 16th June 2000)

Key points

Although philosophical differences have created tension between some religious, spiritual, and faith organizations and victim advocates, common ground can be found in shared interests to end violence against women. What is important in healthcare is that staff recognize the cultural and/or religious values held by the woman and her family, which may impact upon the perception of domestic violence. It is essential that healthcare staff understand that if a woman leaves her abusive partner she may also be sacrificing her way of living, her community and thus an important part of her identity.

Chapter 4

The response of health professionals to domestic violence

Even though almost all women experiencing domestic abuse come into contact with their general practitioner, and many of them with hospital or dental services as a result of their injuries, and/or with mental health services because of the emotional impact of the abuse, very few as yet receive the necessary practical safety advice, continued support or most appropriate support.

(Mullender 1994: 108)

AN HISTORICAL PERSPECTIVE

Studies indicate that often healthcare practitioners have not responded to abused women as well as they might (Williamson 2000: 2–5). As recently as 1999, Harwin, Hague and Malos revealed that in many of the local domestic violence forums, health service representation was frequently non-existent. In some areas health visitors might take an active role, but in the main, doctors and other health personnel rarely took part. More recently, whilst the situation has improved in an increasing number of localities, there remain many healthcare areas where little, if anything, is done to support women abused by intimate partners.

Similar criticism continues to be levelled at social workers, social services, and the civil and criminal justice system, including the police service. Presently, all of these services are having varying degrees of success in their attempts to stem the tide of violence in the home. Mullender (1996) argues that historically social workers have avoided domestic abuse issues unless, or until, dealing with them became a statutory duty directly related to child abuse. Similarly, the police service has frequently been criticized for making minimal, and often ineffectual, responses to what were previously referred to as 'domestic incidents'. Through multi-agency, multi-professional domestic violence forums these individual groups are collectively endeavouring to redress the balance, supporting women and children, and when appropriate men, as they strive to establish a home that is free from violence and abuse.

In recent times, there has been a significant growth in the work undertaken in several healthcare sectors, with an increase in research related to domestic violence and health and a rising number of local and national practice initiatives. It is anticipated that the growth of professional literature, conferences, government initiatives, and publications should compel healthcare personnel across the UK to take an active part in recognizing and facilitating survivors of domestic violence. It is Williamson's belief that in healthcare the growth in concern about domestic violence issues is influenced by a mounting international discourse on women's human rights, and specific health needs. Domestic violence has been designated a major public health issue by both the World Health Organisation and the European Women's Lobby. A number of professional bodies, including the Royal College of Nursing, the Royal College of Midwifery, the British Medical Association and the Royal College of Obstetricians and Gynaecologists, have in the last few years published guidelines related to the management of domestic violence.

WHY DON'T HEALTHCARE PERSONNEL RESPOND TO DOMESTIC VIOLENCE EFFECTIVELY?

> The health service may literally be a lifeline for women whose contact with the outside world is restricted by a violent partner, or who may not wish to become involved with the police or criminal justice system.
>
> (Department of Health [DoH] 2000a: 2)

A range of studies have identified a variety of reasons why we believe healthcare practitioners may not respond as effectively to domestic abuse as they should. Historically, in healthcare institutions the majority of the senior positions, including those of medical personnel, have been held by men, although the majority of the workforce is female. Hence, the lack of commitment to instigating effective policies, procedures and protocols may be a result of men setting the agenda and not perceiving domestic abuse as a public health issue. Traditionally, policy-makers at local, national and international level have been predominantly male and it is therefore not surprising that changes in legislation and government policies on domestic violence have been a long time coming.

Arguably, if one in four women is directly affected by domestic violence, at any one time a significant number of the female employees in the health service are experiencing abuse at home. To avoid confronting the dilemma within their own life, it is not surprising therefore if the individual dealing with the abused client refrains from exploring the client's problem in depth. Equally, if one in four women is abused, and is generally abused by a man, it is feasible that several men within the organization are themselves abusers. If these men were to acknowledge that the client had a problem, then they would either have to ignore the issues or begin to explore and justify their own behaviour.

In a study of medical and nursing staff, including medical students, undertaken in 1996 by DeLahunta and Tulsky, of the 787 respondents, 99 reported physical abuse, sexual abuse, or both by a partner during their adult life. There were 118 who reported physical abuse, sexual abuse, or both, as children, and 188 who reported physical abuse, sexual abuse, or both in their lifetimes. Thus we can see that, based on positive responses, a minimum of 17 per cent of the female medical students and staff, and 3 per cent of the male medical students and staff, had experienced physical abuse or sexual abuse by a partner in their adult life.

Parsons *et al.* (1995: 385) in a study related to domestic violence during pregnancy noted that healthcare practitioners gave the following reasons for not having recognized or intervened in cases of abuse and violence:

- 71 per cent of staff claimed that they failed to intervene due to lack of time
- 55 per cent interviewed said that they feared offending the patient
- 50 per cent reported feelings of inadequacy and frustration in offering appropriate intervention or because they felt they lacked training
- 42 per cent expressed reluctance to intervene as they were unable to control or 'cure' the problem
- staff members, especially female physicians, identified either with the female patient's situation or with her socio-economic status.

The Department of Health (2000a: 20), also suggests that practitioners do not ask the question because they may believe:

- that the woman provoked or 'asked' for it
- that some women deliberately choose violent men
- that domestic violence is not a serious matter or that it is a 'private' one
- that domestic violence is not a healthcare issue.

Other reasons may include:
- it is a waste of time: 'she will only be back'
- it was only a slap, it happens to lots of couples
- 'it is not our business'
- if the victim is male, a disbelief that domestic abuse relates to men or a belief that he probably deserved it
- a male victim may suffer the humiliation of being laughed at and called a wimp, further demoralizing him
- a belief that there is no such thing as marital rape
- the behaviour is 'the norm', it is just the way couples behave
- domestic violence does not happen.

Even today, despite national campaigns, women in violent and abusive relationships suffer the unreal expectations of those providing support services. All too often, the individuals providing services subscribe to the myths identified above.

AVOIDING THE ISSUES

Humphreys's (2000a) study revealed several strategies professionals use to avoid confronting the abuse issues, including:

- supporting the man as the cornerstone of the family rather than challenging his abuse
- inappropriately naming the mother's violence as more of, or as great, a problem as the man's violence towards her
- diverting to other issues such as mental health or alcohol abuse
- ignoring the man altogether in the assessment process, and therefore dismissing any responsibility he has for the violence
- failure to include the domestic violence as a significant issue in the report

- using words and phrases which minimized the degree of violence, e.g. an argument between the parents rather than a violent assault.

Other studies have highlighted that, whilst healthcare workers may feel intervention is appropriate, they do not perceive it to be their business. This may be because staff development is not available and therefore staff do not know how to address the issues. A lack of knowledge and understanding means that staff are frequently unaware of what can be done to help therefore they avoid involving themselves. For example, Tilden *et al.*'s (1994) study found few dentists who considered it to be their business, despite the number of women who suffer broken teeth and jaw injuries. In a few studies, staff have expressed concern for their own safety if they get involved with domestic abuse situations (Davidson *et al.* 2001: 106–7).

Hester *et al.* (2000) indicate a tendency for professionals to categorize domestic violence incidents into a hierarchy of severity according to the degree and severity of physical injury. Even severe emotional and psychological abuse is rated as less severe by professionals, in contrast to the women who suffer at the hands of abusive men, who would argue to the contrary. Therefore, it is possible for the abusive situation to be ignored by the health-worker unless the physical harm to the client is viewed as significant.

Key point

Research has revealed a multiplicity of reasons why healthcare personnel do not 'ask the question', or fail to explore the underlying issues of an assault.
   None is acceptable.

ASKING THE QUESTION

Studies have been undertaken in various healthcare settings to establish how women feel about routine screening for domestic violence. Davidson *et al.* (2001: 95–110), summarizing recent research on domestic abuse, found that generally most women were not averse to being questioned routinely about domestic violence. The women generally agreed that being asked direct questions was preferable to being asked general non-specific questions. Covington (1997), cited in Davidson's work, suggested that women were more likely to disclose if they felt they could trust the person they were talking to. Confidentiality is, not surprisingly, high on the woman's agenda. She fears that her abusive partner may discover she has disclosed details of the abuse to an outsider, especially a professional, which may well cause an escalation in the amount and severity of abuse. Covington *et al.* (1997) found that continuity of care facilitates trust, and therefore disclosure, placing community nurses, midwives, obstetricians, GPs and practice nurses. in a prime position to discover the abuse and to support the client in their choice of intervention.

Overall, the literature indicates that many women are dissatisfied with healthcare interventions as the caregiver often either fails to ask about the abuse or can be dismissive if it is revealed. Furthermore, according to Davidson *et al.* (2001), studies consistently found that failure to undertake routine screening leaves a considerable degree of domestic abuse and violence totally unrecognized.

Key points

By and large, studies have found that:

- Women are often not asked by health professionals about being abused.
- Routine screening of abuse is acceptable provided women can be assured of confidentiality.
- The healthcare giver should be empathetic and not dismissive.
- Women want to be listened to and not judged for staying in the relationship.
- Women would value being given more time to talk to the healthcare practitioner.
- A great deal of abuse remains hidden if routine screening does not take place, leaving women at risk of further injury and even death.

Routine screening has disadvantages, especially if undertaken by untrained staff. The possible consequences of 'opening Pandora's box' for the client, their family, and the health professional could be catastrophic if appropriate support systems are not in place. Education and training for staff and an overview of the literature pertaining to the skills of routine screening are dealt with later in the book.

THE RESPONSE OF PROFESSIONALS TO DOMESTIC VIOLENCE: IMPROVING THE SERVICE

In 1998, the Home Office and the Department of Health began to address the issue of lack of effective healthcare responses on domestic violence, by incorporating health within domestic violence crime reduction initiatives (Williamson 2000: 4). In addition, in 2000, the Department of Health published a resource manual specifically targeting healthcare practitioners at all levels of the organization. The resource manual is based on a series of guidelines published by various healthcare professional bodies including the Royal Colleges and the British Medical Association. First, if care is to improve, all staff throughout healthcare must be aware of the issues related to domestic violence for the clients, their families, and the staff themselves. The principles which cover good practice and are examined in more detail later in the chapter are listed below.

Key points

- It is the responsibility of all healthcare personnel to be aware of the importance of domestic violence.
- A variety of literature, including posters with help-line numbers, must be easily visible in all clinics, wards, surgeries, waiting areas, departments.
- Staff must be aware of the range of options available to the person being abused.
- Local authorities must develop local strategies and guidelines taking multi-agency working into consideration.

- Staff development throughout the service must be implemented with periodic staff updates; this should include how to communicate effectively with the clients to meet their complex needs.
- Staff development should also focus on interviewing techniques and intervention.
- Each department and speciality should have its own protocols and advice sheets for staff related to domestic violence as it pertains to their area, e.g. Accident and Emergency, obstetrics and gynaecology, orthopaedics, mental health, community and public health services.
- Supportive information should be made available to clients in a variety of languages to suit the needs of the local population.
- Similarly, a list of interpreters should be available, as it may be inappropriate for a woman to be supported by a close family member or a friend.
- There is a need for more comprehensive research into the health aspects of domestic abuse, including costs, effective interventions, and the efficacy of multi-agency working.

The responsibility of the organization: putting domestic violence on the agenda

To be successful, where possible strategies should be implemented across the organization simultaneously rather than in an ad hoc manner to ensure the client is to be offered continuity of care. Furthermore, staff required to implement care in this area need to feel supported and adequately prepared to deal with the multiplicity of issues which arise when dealing with a client abused in an intimate relationship. The organization must provide comprehensive guidelines for the complex challenges that each staff member might face.

Domestic violence and the workplace

The stress of working in the 'caring professions' is well documented, as is the fact that often organizations do not provide adequate support for their own staff. If, as the DoH insists, all healthcare professionals are to raise their awareness for dealing with clients who are being subjected to domestic violence, arguably the organization must first support and protect its own staff.

It was noted earlier that within all areas of health and social care, a significant proportion of the workforce is female, and at some point in their life many of these women experience abuse and violence within the home. However, research reveals that few employing organizations, including health organizations, in the United Kingdom have domestic violence policies related to staff in place. This section explores the need for all employers, including health providers, to implement policies and procedures that support, and in some instances protect, staff abused in the home.

Domestic violence does not stay home when its victims go to work. It can follow them, resulting in violence in the workplace. Or it can spill over into the workplace

when a woman is harassed by threatening phone calls, absent because of injuries or
less productive from extreme stress.

(GMB 2000)

It should be noted that this section focuses on the woman; however, most of what is
included is equally relevant to men if they are being abused. In addition, men might find
it difficult to disclose abuse as it is often met with ridicule and further abuse from friends
and colleagues. Some of the trade unions and organizations have addressed this by
making policies gender-neutral.

When considering how domestic violence can affect people in the workplace a number
of issues exist. First, the individual being abused may find concentrating on the job in hand
extremely difficult because of the trauma that may be occurring at home. In a work-
shop run at the Trades Union Congress (TUC) Annual Women's Conference in 2000
an attempt was made to highlight what the issues were for women in the workplace.
Their deliberations concluded that the main issues were related to the following aspects.

Performance in the workplace

The delegates agreed with studies that showed that women are often unable to concen-
trate or complete their designated workload because of the emotional and psychological
trauma suffered in their personal life. These factors can affect women's pay, conditions
and benefits, especially where pay is performance-related. Furthermore, the trade union
movement believes that in the long term this could affect the women's career progress
and job opportunities, especially if they needed to leave employment to escape a violent
partner. Furthermore, the abused person may have to take sickness leave if the physical
injuries are moderate to severe. Others require time off to deal with, for example, legal
proceedings, or visits to the social services or housing advisory agencies. An organization
that has not made a definitive statement, or implemented policies supporting staff who
are being victimized in the home, makes it difficult for individuals to disclose the reason
for needing time off.

Confidentiality

. . . a real or perceived lack of confidentiality in the workplace means many women
continue to suffer in silence which in turn perpetuates the invisibility of the crime.
(TUC Annual Women's Conference 2002)

Women have expressed concern that if they divulge their personal circumstances to their
employers, confidentiality is not always guaranteed. A particular problem arises if the
couple works in the same organization and the perpetrator has direct or indirect access
to the victim's personal file. This apprehension may continue even after the woman
leaves the company, as new employers are likely to ask for references which continue to
be kept in the woman's personal file. Where the person being abused is in a homosexual
relationship, fear that the relationship may be disclosed is another major worry; the
threat of 'outing' a person is a strategy commonly used by abusers to control their partners.

In addition, the conference participants noted that women who were home-workers, were agency workers, or worked in isolated areas were likely to have greater difficulty accessing help. They also noted that

> Where there was a 'gender imbalance' in the workplace and it was very male dominated, or the workplace had a 'macho culture' such as the military, police, prison service, women could find it hard to talk about their experiences or develop informal networks.
>
> (TUC Annual Women's Conference 2002)

Cost to the employer

According to the GMB union, there has been little if any academic research carried out in this country to identify the potential cost of domestic violence to industry. However, they found that a recent New York study produced the following statistics.

- 56 per cent of victims were late for work at least five times a month
- 28 per cent had to leave early at least five days a month
- 54 per cent missed at least three full days of work per month.

Individuals being subjected to domestic violence often:

- demonstrate an increase in sickness absence
- demonstrate a decrease in productivity
- demonstrate poor work performance
- may require 'special time' for attendances at court, etc.

The potential role of the trade unions

> Domestic violence is a trade union issue. All violence against women, whether it happens at work, at home or in the community, is a legitimate concern for trade unionists. The effects of domestic violence can be far-reaching. Home and work issues cannot always be separated, and domestic violence can therefore have an impact on job performance, threatening job prospects, and security. It threatens the health of sufferers. It threatens lives.
>
> (Public and Commercial Services Union [PCSU], UK)

The Health and Safety at Work Act 1974 states quite clearly that all employers have a 'duty of care' to their employees in relation to personal safety in the workplace. Whilst there is no direct reference to domestic violence within the Act, nevertheless many unions are now stressing the need for employers to implement policies related to domestic violence issues. The policies need to address issues related to the individual suffering the abuse, but more recently, some companies are recognizing the potential threat posed when domestic violence spills into the workplace.

POLICIES AND PRACTICES THAT MAKE A DIFFERENCE

Guide to good practice

A review of the literature from the UK and the USA suggests that the following elements should be included when designing workplace policies and procedures related to domestic violence. However, the size of the organization may dictate what is achievable in terms of practical assistance.

Raising awareness amongst all staff

Literature must be available so that staff at all levels of the organization are aware of the essential facts related to abuse and violence in the home. This may be achieved by providing posters, information sheets, staff development, workshops, articles in in-company publications, etc. The organization should appoint a designated department or individual to ensure that the information is readily available and up-to-date. Literature must also be made available for those who need direct help; this should include information related to:

- what help is available and where it can be found
- emergency help-line numbers
- local refuges
- local and national support organizations such as Women's Aid
- police contact numbers
- legal services
- useful web pages.

Good practice

PCSU includes in its guidelines aspects that organizations need to consider for inclusion in their policies in relation to abusive situations:

- job flexibility, as well as paid special leave, in case there is a need for the person being abused to work irregular hours
- ensuring there is no penalization through scrutiny of sick leave
- support if redeployment is requested at no cost to the woman, ensuring her new working location is not revealed
- a clause on job security and stating that inefficiency procedures are not instigated
- pay should not be affected by adverse appraisal markings if women are unable to function effectively.

Staff development

Depending on the size of the organization, managers need to consider the potential for training managers or designated personnel in aspects of domestic abuse including:

- designing effective policies

- supporting staff who are being abused at home including how to ask the questions and offer effective support. This can be a skilful and emotionally draining role so those undertaking it require appropriate training and support.
- workshops for team members where appropriate
- some staff may need to become familiar with legal aspects of violence, including Health and Safety at Work policies and the implication of domestic violence.

Key point

All healthcare organizations, including trade unions allied to healthcare, must be seen to be supporting their own staff, if healthcare professionals are to make a difference to their clients.

Therefore, staff charged with writing the policies and procedures to protect clients may wish to enter a dialogue with their own employers about the health and welfare of the staff.

WHEN THE VIOLENCE ENTERS THE WORKPLACE

Unless and until those who run organizations familiarize themselves with the threat of domestic violence in the workplace, exposure to such a threat may become a reality.
(American Federation of State, County and Municipal Employees [AFSCME] last updated 2000)

There is a growing concern in the United States, and more recently in the United Kingdom, about how workers are put at risk when a violent man seeks out his female (or male) partner at work. When domestic violence spills over into the workplace, the outcomes are unpredictable and the consequences can be fatal. The US Department of Justice estimates that husbands and boyfriends commit 13,000 acts of violence against women in the workplace every year.

A few private employers and state governments have taken steps to address domestic violence at work. In 1996, the governor of Washington ordered each state agency and higher educational institution to develop policies and procedures to assist victims of domestic violence.

(AFSCME 2000)

Keeping staff safe

Ensure a safe working environment by taking all reasonable steps to guard against the threat of domestic violence, which may carry over into the workplace.

(GMB 2000)

Apart from the general guidelines related to health and safety at work, few policies in the United Kingdom appear to offer specific staff safety guidelines related to domestic violence. With the significant increase in violence against healthcare staff, general policies and procedures in relation to dealing with violence have been employed. With a few additions, these guidelines could perhaps highlight the specific aspects of violence related to domestic violence.

In the United States, where there have been a number of recorded incidents of serious injury and even fatal injury, existing guides suggest that organizations should:

- encourage management to enhance security in the workplace to prohibit the victim's abuser (and other non-employees) from entering the work area unescorted
- provide advance warning and photographs to security guards and workers in the building about the danger posed by the victim's abuser. This of course has implications for the confidentiality of the individual staff member, who might then be required to notify employers of the potential risk.
- ensure a safe working environment by taking all reasonable steps to guard against the threat of domestic violence, which may carry over into the workplace.

(GMB 2000)

For healthcare institutions, it is vital they implement support and guidance for their own staff on how to care for themselves as well as clients.

WRITING PROTOCOLS AND POLICIES

Each healthcare organization including trusts, primary care trusts or private hospital services ought to begin by designing widespread policies and procedures that include a comprehensive staff development programme to raise awareness. The DoH (2000a: 41) advises that policies and protocols should be developed and tested in consultation with different stakeholder groups. Practice guidelines should include 'interview technique and principles to be followed; and action following disclosure'. Each health organization has a responsibility either to establish links with an existing multi-agency domestic violence forum, or, where none exists, to take responsibility for setting one up. Local, regional and national health organizations need to establish an effective networking system to avoid re-inventing the wheel.

Perhaps this is an opportune moment for professional bodies to work together to provide a comprehensive and collective set of guidelines which highlight the need for multi-disciplinary, multi-agency co-operation. Historically, health and social care professionals may have had different, and occasionally contradictory, philosophies, priorities, protocols and guidelines that may have militated against a harmonious and effective collaborative process. For this reason, many organizations are calling for far greater multi-agency, multi-disciplinary practice in the area of domestic violence.

The first step: defining domestic violence

Chapter 1 highlighted some of the strengths and potential weaknesses of specific rather than generic definitions of domestic violence and abuse. When dealing with domestic violence in an area as broad as healthcare, unless certain groups are to be discriminated against, the definition needs to be all-encompassing.

Key points

Any definition of domestic violence and abuse must address the key factors:

- A definition should recognize all the groups that may be abused in an intimate relationship including women, men and transgender individuals, and couples in same-sex relationships. However, it must be acknowledged that the majority of the abuse is male on female, in an intimate relationship.
- A definition must recognize the power and control aspects which underpins the abuse.
- The definition should be clear about which groups are included. It may be more appropriate to have separate guidelines for the elderly or disabled clients as they may be subject to significant abuse from non-intimate individuals as well.
- It must identify the range of abuse, including physical, psychological, financial, emotional, and sexual.
- It may be appropriate to include the historical, social and political influences that underpin domestic abuse.
- It might also include a statement about the effects on children of living in a home where intimate abuse exists.
- Where appropriate, separate guidelines may need to be developed for the safety and welfare of children in an abusive home.

Once the definition has been agreed key personnel can begin to set the agenda and embark on designing policies and procedures.

Staff roles and responsibilities

It is essential that the roles and responsibilities of individuals and groups within the organization are identified and defined. Senior staff, such as department heads, have over-arching responsibilities, whereas the focus for the individual practitioner is directly on individual client care. Some health organizations are appointing staff with specialist knowledge to take the agenda forward. It may be appropriate to link with the local higher education provider, or one of the national domestic violence organizations such as the Women's Aid Federation, for guidance.

Any organizational policies should, wherever possible, acknowledge and articulate with the role of other agencies such as the legal services, social services, and housing and voluntary agencies, including the women's refuge centre. It is essential that the relationship between the agencies and the healthcare organization be articulated. Staff may require guidance as to, for example, confidentiality. At some time in the future, patient notes may be used in a criminal prosecution and therefore staff need to know their legal responsibilities in such matters.

Confidentiality

All healthcare staff are familiar with the professional and legal requirement pertaining to client confidentiality. Nevertheless, this aspect of care must be emphasized in any guidelines, as the life and liberty of the person being abused may be in jeopardy from their current or ex-partner. The BMA (1999) advise that confidentiality should be discussed with the client on each occasion that the issue of domestic violence is raised. The essence of the advice should be that confidentiality will be maintained at all times. However, the health professional must make it clear to the client disclosing that there are rare circumstances, such as where children are potentially at risk from harm, where silence may not be possible. Equally, it may be impossible to maintain confidentiality if the woman is contemplating self-harm, or the injuries have been severe, and the continuing threat to the woman is judged potentially fatal.

This aspect of confidentiality may have implications for the client disclosing. She is unlikely to continue the consultation if she fears that the child welfare services, or the police service, may be involved, and thus the option of utilizing outside intervention is no longer under her control. It may have taken a great deal of courage for the woman to admit to the violence she has suffered; withdrawing at this stage is undoubtedly detrimental to her future health and well-being and that of any children.

Whilst doctors are bound by the code of conduct as defined by the General Medical Council (GMC), nurses, midwives and health visitors would be required to comply with their professional Code of Conduct which states that:

> 5.3 You must treat information about patients and clients as confidential and use it only for the purposes for which it was given. As it is impractical to obtain consent every time you need to share information with others, you should ensure that patients and clients understand that some information may be made available to other members of the team involved in the delivery of care. You must guard against breaches of confidentiality by protecting information from improper disclosure at all times.
> 5.4 Where there is an issue of child protection, you must act at all times in accordance with national and local policies.
> (Nursing and Midwifery Council, Code of Professional Conduct 2002)

The Department of Health (2002a: 38) offers broad advice to healthcare professionals in relation to confidentiality as it specifically relates to domestic violence. The DoH agrees that confidentiality in such cases, especially where children are involved, can be complex and that healthcare professionals must work together and with others to prevent confidentiality being inadvertently breached. The department illustrates the potential dilemmas by giving as an example the possibility of a child from a refuge being admitted to hospital. In the event of the father visiting, it is essential that information related to the family's current living location must not, under any circumstances, be disclosed. Where the health professional such as a practice nurse, GP, community nurse or health visitor is working with the whole family, it is essential that confidentiality is not breached.

The BMA and the DoH, as well as the Nursing and Midwifery Council (NMC) in its Code of Professional Conduct, emphasize the care that should be taken when disclosing confidential information. Each trust, PCT, or private hospital would therefore be advised to have in place comprehensive guidelines, policies and procedures as appropriate. Staff should be strongly advised to discuss the case before making a definitive judgement about disclosure. The issues related specifically to confidentiality, disclosure, domestic abuse, and children are to be covered in more detail in Chapter 7. Overarching and examples of good practice are addressed in Chapter 5.

This chapter has highlighted the need for healthcare professionals and organizations to act in a co-ordinated way, ensuring that staff and clients are adequately informed and supported and that safety is maintained at all times. The following chapter addresses specific areas in which good practice is imperative.

Chapter 5

A critique of existing healthcare provision

Experts in the field of domestic abuse and healthcare provision, generally agree that one of the challenges to improving the response to clients is the continued use by the professionals of a medical model of care framework. The violence and abuse are frequently reduced by the professional to a physical, psychological or mental health diagnosis and treatment, without due consideration given to the social and political location of violence. In effect, such an approach locates the 'problem' in the individuals sustaining the injuries or presenting with the ill-health aftermath of years of abuse. The clients are 'treated' according to their signs and symptoms and often left feeling as though either the problem is theirs, or alternatively that she or he is the problem.

> [The] medical approach reduces male violence – a social process rooted in gender identity – to biological, individual or situational factors and focuses prevention on the individual level. This focus minimises the historical and social dimensions of women's experiences that are so crucial to understanding and responding appropriately to wife-battery. Clinicians learn to catalogue abuse alongside other 'illnesses'. Whether abused women are received like other patients requiring 'treatment' or as 'victims' requiring 'rescue', medical interventions inevitably reproduce and extend female dependence.
>
> (Kurz and Stark 1988: 262)

Stark and Flitcraft (1996) advocate a fundamental change in the current philosophical approach of healthcare provision when dealing with the consequences of domestic abuse. Health professionals must recognize that the issues go far beyond the individual requiring 'treatment', they have to acknowledge and challenge the wider political, social and gender constructs which frame our existing interpretations of family violence.

In 1999 Abbott and Williamson undertook an important study to identify the strengths and weaknesses of existing healthcare provision as it relates to domestic abuse in the UK. The study explored the views of members of a community health team, including GPs, health visitors, practice nurses and midwives, of a specific healthcare provider.

> The role that healthcare professionals can play is severely limited by their lack of knowledge and understanding. They are not well equipped to empower women and enable them to make informed decisions. . . . Working within the dominant bio-medical model, they individualise the cause, medicalising what is a social problem –

they treat the specific biological problem. This reinforces the powerlessness of women and the medical control of them . . . reinforcing dependency and compliance.

(Abbott and Williamson 1999: 4)

This insight is particularly relevant to members of the medical profession who, according to the BMA, are traditionally educated into the medical model of care. 'This model focuses on objectivity and placing patients in a diagnostic category for which there is defined treatment . . . [And] may result in the true cause of the woman's symptoms being obscured' (British Medical Association [BMA] 1999: 38). Abbott and Williamson (1999) discovered that it was health visitors, used to working in close contact and collaboration with social workers, who were less likely to adopt the medical-model approach. However, a criticism of their methods was that generally their primary concern, perhaps not surprisingly, was the health and safety of any children in the home.

Stevens (1997) believes that the healthcare professionals' definition of 'a successful intervention' may require some modification, as their perception of 'success' and the clients' may differ significantly. Leaving a violent relationship is, as we have already discovered, often a process. However, a single encounter with a member of the healthcare team may ultimately have an important impact for the woman at some point in the future. Being given the telephone number of a help line may be in itself sufficient to support the woman at a future date.

One way health providers can move towards a non-medical model of practice is to ensure that policies, practices and procedures are informed by a knowledge and consideration of the work being done in multi-agency forums. Only then can the health disciplines recognize the far wider implications of abuse within intimate relationships. 'There is a serious problem with domestic violence being relegated to a position of secondary diagnosis rather than being perceived as the cause of the injury requiring a primary diagnosis of its own' (Williamson 2000: 23). Williamson (2000) argues that within the medical framework currently used, health professionals often relegate domestic violence to a secondary diagnosis rather than making it the primary diagnosis. It is worthy of note that in a health service increasingly based on clinical specialities there are few recognized 'specialist' consultants in domestic abuse and violence, despite the fact that the Department of Health, the World Health Organisation, and most of the professional bodies for health practitioners have designated domestic violence a major public health issue.

Nevertheless, it remains an imperative for healthcare personnel to continue to distinguish and act upon the physical, psychological and mental health aspects of an individual's situation. Specific aspects of care are discussed in detail in Chapter 6, addressing the role and responsibilities of various clinical health specialities. Williamson argues that to ignore the violence as the primary diagnosis relegates it to a set of signs and symptoms, which, treated separately, discount the lived-in reality of the women who experience it. If the primary diagnosis is a fractured skull, the need for legal, social and political intervention is easily overlooked.

> **Key point**
>
> Where a client seeks help medical assistance for an event directly related to abuse and violence from an intimate partner, a clinical diagnosis of a physical or psychological condition alone does not suffice. To be effective, assessment and care management must be based on and reflect the seriousness of the overarching domestic abuse and its wider ramifications.

EMPOWERMENT AS A STRATEGY FOR MOVING FORWARD

> Health professionals assist in a process of empowerment and self-management by the woman of her situation, and it may be some time before she is ready to take definitive action.
>
> (British Medical Association [BMA] 1999)

Where there has been criticism of healthcare practices and domestic violence, it has often focused around a lack of understanding of the woman's needs. Often, as we saw earlier, the question in many people's minds is 'Why doesn't she leave?' and the response to the woman who continually puts up with the abuse may be less than supportive. Abbott and Williamson's study (1999) clearly demonstrated that health professionals within the UK generally do not have a comprehensive awareness of many of the issues underpinning violence within intimate relationships. It is therefore not surprising that their ability to respond effectively is limited by a lack of knowledge and understanding of the subject.

To be successful in the long term, the focus of care must be on empowering the woman to make her own choices and to do what she feels is necessary at a time which is right for her. Empowerment, according to many writers can only be achieved when the client has sufficient knowledge and skills to both make and carry out her own wishes. For the woman being abused, knowing what assistance is 'out there', knowing who to talk to and what can be done enables her to make choices which are valid for her and her children. The healthcare professionals should accept that this takes time and that therefore their role may be one of support, acting as an adviser, as a resource and, on occasions, as an advocate.

Healthcare professionals, alongside the other members of the multi-agency team, can individually and collectively, over time, offer the woman both the advice and the necessary assistance to make her survival a reality at a time to suit her.

> The single most empowering thing any practitioner can offer a woman who is being abused is to take her seriously and to assist her to become safe, in whatever way she feels best to her when she considers her own and her children's needs and knows the options available.
>
> (Mullender 1996: 266)

A framework for empowerment

Mullender (1996: 267 and 275) offers a framework for empowerment originally for use by social workers; however, this could be easily adapted for healthcare professionals supporting a client in an abusive relationship. First, the woman needs to be believed. She needs to know that the individual she is talking to is not sitting in judgement, and she needs to be confident that if she does not take his or her advice this time, if she returns she will receive care which is non-judgemental and in her best interest.

Key points

Mullender (1996) advocates important principles needed to underpin any care offered. The following important points incorporate these principles as they could be applied to healthcare.

- Any woman seeking help should be viewed with respect, as an individual possessing sufficient strength to survive, who already has skills, understanding, and abilities.
- Like all women, she has rights; particularly the right to choose her own pathway without incurring negative responses by those from whom she seeks help. 'She is the expert in his dangerousness and on her own safety' (Mullender 1996: 275).
- The health professional should not seek to explain either the abuser's or the abused person's situation and behaviour simply in terms of personal inadequacies, as to do so denies the important context of social and gender inequalities.

The recognition of domestic violence as a social problem – a political as opposed to a personal issue – has yet to become the norm, and until this fact is accepted by all professionals, organizations, etc. rather than individualizing the problem, interventions will be limited and do little to empower the women.

(Abbott and Williamson 1999: 6)

Key points

- The health professional must recognize that without other agencies offering appropriate services simultaneously, the woman is unlikely to be successful if she exits the relationship. Personal health and safety are often dependent upon having somewhere safe to stay, being protected by law, being financially independent and being free from fear.
- Mullender emphasizes the important role that is played by women's support groups. The significance of the role of the women's refuge is well documented and readers are advised to access some of the resources identified at the end of the book. Many women's refuges offer access to support groups to women who have not needed to use the residential facilities, and many continue to offer support long after the woman leaves. Mullender (1996: 275) believes that a group in which the participants find solutions collectively is one of the most empowering and therefore effective creations possible.
- By operating within a multi-disciplinary, multi-agency framework, healthcare professionals can have a major voice in the professional, political and social discourse needed for domestic abuse to be located on local, national and international agendas.

MEETING THE CHALLENGE IN HEALTHCARE PROVISION

A UK-wide study, *From Good Intentions to Good Practice: a Mapping Study of Services working with Families where there is Domestic Violence*, was carried out in 1999, to establish the range and extent of domestic violence service provision across the country. The study was supported by the Joseph Rowntree Foundation. Following on from this report, a *Good Practice Guide* has been authored by Humphreys, Hague, Hester and Mullender, and published by the University of Warwick. Details of how to access the full report and a copy of the Good Practice Indicators can be found in the resource section at the end of the book. Each of these aspects of good practice is covered in various chapters of this book.

The *Good Practice Indicators* include:

1: *The Use of Definitions of Domestic Violence*
2: *The Use of Monitoring Processes and Screening*
3: *Good Practice Guidelines and Domestic Violence Policies*
4: *Safety Planning*
5: *Training*
6: *Evaluation*
7: *Multi-Agency Integration and Co-ordination*
8: *Working with Women and Children*

As we noted in Chapter 2, the first step for any organization or department is to define the subject. For healthcare the most appropriate format might be to have a wider organizational definition covering the diverse client and staff group spectrum, and for departments to adapt this where necessary for their specific client group. For example, the definition in a midwifery unit may differ from that being used in a men's self-help group. Similarly, the focus of assessment and care delivery should be modified according to the specific clinical setting. For instance, mental health units may have a different focus than an Accident and Emergency unit, regarding clients' mental health needs. In the latter, the focus is liable to be on immediate needs, whereas a mental health specialist unit as a rule focuses on short-, medium- and long-term facilitation.

According to Humphreys, an acceptable overarching definition might be one that is gender-neutral, whilst acknowledging the fact that most abuse is on a woman by a known male. The definition should be inclusive and acknowledge diversity:

> Definitions need to include different types of abuse (e.g. physical, emotional, sexual etc.) and to recognize diversity of experience. The best definitions recognize the wide-ranging effects of domestic violence and the fact that it may have impacts on children in the family.
>
> (Humphreys *et al.* 2001: 4)

Equally, the definition should indicate the nature of the violence by locating it within a power and coercion framework.

Routine screening

How and when to ask about domestic violence is a difficult and emotive issue which may feel intrusive. However, carefully developed and sensitive procedural guidelines, routinely used by all staff, are of help. Systematic routine screening is vital (but universal screening is a complex issue and needs to be developed with care).

(Humphreys *et al.* 2000: 2)

Routine screening is defined by the Family Violence Prevention Fund (FVPF) as

Routine inquiry, either written or verbal, by healthcare providers to patients about personal history with domestic violence. Unlike indicator based screening, routine screening means screening conducted routinely on all individuals or specified categories of individuals in a specified situation.

As yet, there is no consensus amongst health professionals about routine screening, with the debate focusing around questions such as should screening be routine and standard and if so, by whom should it be carried out and how should it be done. The evidence from survivors as we saw earlier is generally positive; many expressed the view that they wished someone had asked the question. The physician's concern about abuse validates the woman's feelings and reinforces her capacity to seek help when she feels ready and able to do so (AMA 1992). However, studies from professionals are not as conclusive, with many staff expressing a reluctance to involve themselves in the process.

The professional health bodies in the UK have not yet made a definitive statement about whether or not screening should be obligatory in healthcare. Interestingly, the Royal College of Nursing's *Domestic Violence: Guidance for Nurses* (2000) cover a number of care aspects but omit any discussion of routine screening. The BMA (1999: 41) confirms that British guidelines implemented in healthcare settings are not common and tends to shy away from recommending routine questioning. According to the DoH (March 2000: 23), the Health Services Circular HSC 1988/211, which followed the 'Confidential Report into Maternal Deaths' (1988), states quite clearly the need for 'routine questioning in ante-natal care, and sensitive enquiry about domestic violence being included in taking a social history'.

Jane Morgan (2002) at the annual meeting of the Royal College of Midwives (RCM) noted that the debate about the degree of involvement needed by practising midwives in relation to domestic violence is far from decided. The Royal College of Midwives has published a position paper, which includes advice about client assessment of domestic violence but yet does not require midwives to undertake routine screening.

The RCM recommends that every midwife assumes a role in the detection and management of domestic abuse, given its damaging impact on the outcome of pregnancy. Every midwife has a responsibility to provide each woman in her care with support, information and referral appropriate to her needs.

(Royal College of Midwives 1999)

Heath (2000) authored a guide for the Royal College of General Practitioners on recognition and management of patients who are, or have been, in an abusive relationship.

Within the guide, GPs are advised to consider routine screening and the types of questions which might be appropriate.

The DoH (2000: 24) advocates the introduction of routine screening in all areas of healthcare, with the proviso that:

> Routine questioning about domestic violence *must* be accompanied by appropriate protocols, and training and support for all staff involved. Approaches to routine enquiry should employ validated screening questions and methodologies. . . . Routine screening should not be treated as a 'one-off' episode.

Key point

Whilst many healthcare professionals agree that routine screening is an important healthcare process not everyone concurs. However, there is little point in screening unless appropriate follow-up support systems are in place. Acknowledging, or alerting a woman to the fact that she is in an abusive situation, without then offering her assistance would be both inappropriate and potentially harmful. All healthcare staff must be adequately trained to deal with clients who are enduring domestic abuse, and have access to the literature to support staff and clients provided by the health authority. Moreover, health professionals must be working in collaboration with other agencies expert in domestic violence and abuse.

Benefits of routine screening include:

- Women in a variety of studies welcomed the routine screening (Taylor-Browne 2001: 109–12).
- It ensures staff at all levels are involved within the process, particularly where the screening is extended into the role of the nurses as well as of medics.
- Depending upon what questions are asked it may help the individual to recognize that she is in an abusive relationship.
- It can support women by making them realize that it is a situation shared by many other individuals, so that they know they are not alone.
- When the questioning is supported by information packs, posters, help lines and other information it may highlight the fact that sometimes solutions are possible.

Taylor-Browne (2001: 109), having undertaken a comprehensive review of healthcare literature, provides a useful summary of the major studies that relate directly to routine screening for domestic abuse. Like other authors (Mullender 1996; Humphreys 2001c), Taylor-Browne concluded that routine screening is only effective when accompanied by appropriate staff training and development. As well, the organization needs to have in place validated screening tools for effective care, for evaluative studies to be undertaken and for future auditing of the process. Without an established screening instrument and a departmental commitment to routine screening, assessment remains ad hoc and is likely to leave many clients at risk.

However, a recent study undertaken at Queen Mary's Hospital in London, advises that, as yet, we have insufficient evidence to support routine screening across the UK without further work being done. In particular the authors conclude that the following research questions need to be answered before healthcare professionals can be confident that routine screening is appropriate.

Research questions

- What are the benefits and risks to women of screening for domestic violence in health-care settings?
- What is the most effective screening interval?
- What is the effect of participation in interventions such as provision of advocacy support on women experiencing domestic violence identified in healthcare settings?
- What are the training needs of health professionals in relation to domestic violence?
- How can we promote better multi-agency working in this area?

(Ramsay et al. 2000)

Clinical and nursing assessment

Depending upon the circumstances of the health assessment the practitioner undertaking the assessment should be on the alert for physical signs of injury as identified in Chapter 2. In addition, it may be appropriate to question the clients about their general state of health including sleeping patterns, signs of excessive tiredness and signs of hyper-vigilance (when the client flinches easily; constantly appears to be on the alert for possible danger; is nervous, and over-anxious). The client may show signs of depression and/or anxiety and of exceedingly low self-esteem. Equally, psychologically and emotionally, the woman may appear quite capable of controlling her own destiny, but it does not mean that she is not being seriously abused and/or assaulted by her partner.

ASSESSMENT: ASKING THE QUESTION

A detailed discussion on the appropriate way to undertake routing screening and the types of questions that might be asked is covered later. It is imperative that staff involved in the assessment process undergo suitable training in what questions to ask and how to carry out the assessment. In order that they can offer effective client care, staff need to feel confident that they are adequately prepared. Where individual staff members develop a degree of expertise in this area, they may well find that supporting clients in domestic abuse situations becomes a primary role function. In such cases, it would be advisable for such persons to have regular access to clinical supervision, ensuring that they are supported at all times.

Creating a safe environment

One of the challenges of questioning a patient who is being abused is finding a safe space in which to ask the questions. Often in an abusive relationship the partner stays by the client's side, sometimes answering for them and making it extremely difficult for a rapport to develop between the client and staff. Asking the partner to leave may, of course, allow the professional to ask the necessary questions; however, staff should remember that the partner will undoubtedly interrogate the client once they leave the building. Therefore, the client's safety must remain the overwhelming priority throughout the assessment and intervention processes. Care should be taken when excluding the partner from the consultation; this is particularly important in midwifery care when there is normally an expectation that visits to the midwife are with both partners where possible.

Similarly, any information given to the client such as X-ray forms, blood forms, and referral letters should not indicate that the possibility of abuse is being considered. Where notes are kept, confidentiality is of paramount importance and it may be necessary for organizations and departments to establish specific protocols for the safe keeping of records.

Key point

Where a client with a health need possibly caused by domestic abuse, is unable to speak adequate English, care should be taken to find an interpreter. Often when clients are unable to speak the language a member of the family or close friend acts as interpreter. In a situation where domestic abuse is suspected this might prevent the woman from speaking out; alternatively what she is actually saying may not be interpreted correctly to the health staff. Staff of course must take great care; finding an interpreter can take time and any unnecessary delay may be viewed by the woman's partner with suspicion. When staff deal with a client whom they suspect is in an abusive relationship, maintaining the immediate safety of that client is of paramount importance.

Record-keeping

It is possible that having dealt with a client with injuries as a result of violence from an intimate partner, staff may be required to give evidence to a court of law. Therefore, a full and accurate record of the patient's history and treatment, and of advice offered should be made at the time. Similarly, if there are any altercations in the clinical setting involving the patient's partner, it may be appropriate to complete an incident form. The DoH (2000a) emphasizes the need for full and accurate documentation, pointing out that these records may be the means whereby a woman can gain an injunction against the abusive partner.

Health records related to domestic abuse may need to be kept separate from those being held by a patient or which the perpetrator could have access to. This includes taking care when giving forms, e.g. for X-ray consultations, not to indicate possible cause of injury. Keeping accurate records is essential and should, as appropriate, include:

- an accurate account of the history as given by the patient/client
- an accurate record of all physical injuries, preferably using a diagrammatic body map
- signs of old injury or injuries including bruises, scars and healed fractures
- signs of impaired mental or emotional well-being
- signs of gynaecological problems or injury, which might have been acquired as a result of aggressive sexual activity. (Any such signs might be a result of non-consensual sex, and may have implications for any criminal charges made against the perpetrator.)

- Where possible, photographic evidence should be obtained. The woman may be advised to have photographs taken for her own records, particularly if on this occasion she is not involving the police services. (See Appendix 7.)
- It is imperative that any records kept must *not* be accessible to the abuser. This is particularly important in areas such as midwifery, where the patient keeps her personal records.
- Where appropriate, records should incorporate reports from members of the multi-disciplinary team and should indicate clearly details of any referrals and follow-up appointments.

Policies and protocols

According to Humphreys *et al.* (2000), any organizational policies should:

- Ensure that the refuge movement and related women's support and advocacy projects retain a central role. The Women's Aid movement along with other groups have exceptional expertise in all areas of domestic violence, therefore their views and input are imperative.
- *Pay attention to diversity, equality, and consultation with survivors.* Not all organizational policy-makers take the 'user's' perspective into consideration. Who could know better than a 'survivor' what may or may not work? If we are writing policies to include the needs of, for example, ethnic minority groups or women with disabilities, their views should inform practice.
- *Work together within a wider strategy across a locality.* Health organizations alone can achieve little progress. To be successful they need to collaborate with other agencies and organizations; where more than one organization is involved, policies need to be complementary to one another.
- *Develop a broad range of policies and guidelines and clarity in the referral system.* The Good Practice Guidelines point out that any policies must recognize the specific needs of different client groups, including policies for the health and well-being of children, of individuals with disabilities, perpetrators and others. 'Issues covered may include staff safety procedures, information for service users and detailed practical guidelines for front line workers' (Humphreys *et al.* 2000: 6).
- The guidelines specify there is little point in re-inventing the wheel. Tried and tested procedures and protocols successfully used by other organizations can be used as a basis for new work.

Policies and procedures are of little use unless, and until, they become a part of the organization's norms. A comprehensive staff development programme must be put into effect across the organization prior to policy implementation. Such programmes need to continue on a regular basis if the policies are to become embedded within the institution's operational practice. A more detailed exploration of staff development programmes is covered later in the book.

Providing information

Studies have shown that one of the major reasons why women are unable to leave a violent and abusive relationship is that they do not know how to take the first step. Often they have been isolated from friends and from families and the shame of sharing their situation with an 'outsider' is too great. Moreover, the women often feel there is nothing that can be done anyway, or that their only option is to leave their home and go to a refuge. However, if the children are not being physically abused, the woman may be reluctant to take this action thinking that it would be a retrograde step for them.

One of the important ways that healthcare personnel can make a difference is by providing a variety of literature to both staff and the members of the public. Organizations such as the Women's Aid Federation, or the local police services, often through the local multi-agency domestic violence forum, provide a comprehensive set of literature for clients. With the advent of the Internet, materials are readily available for the individual being abused, for any member of the public with an interest in the subject, and for the healthcare worker. Visitors to many of the Internet sites are given clear instructions on how to keep themselves safe. However, using the Internet can leave behind an easy-to-follow trail on the computer's history, so sites give instructions on how to delete this.

Handing out literature to women in clinics, Accident and Emergency departments and other healthcare venues may put the woman at risk, especially if she has been accompanied by her violent partner. Staff therefore need to assess the potential risk to the client. One of the safest places to situate information is within the ladies' toilet, as it is the one location few men would consider entering. It is possible to purchase small stickers with an emergency help-line number on, which can be placed on the back of the door of the toilet cubicle. Displaying posters with help-line numbers around the building can be a powerful way to put the message across. If it can be seen that the subject of domestic violence is a general health concern, then the perpetrator may be less suspicious if his partner is questioned. Suggestions that are more specific are offered in the chapter dealing with different healthcare settings.

Healthcare providers need to seek innovative ways of spreading the message first to the staff who are dealing with clients in abusive relationships and second to those who are being abused. Perhaps more importantly the work must be continuous; staff development should persist over time possibly becoming mandatory. Periodic local and national campaigns also have to be organized; the public requires a greater awareness of the help available for those living in abusive relationships.

RISK ASSESSMENT AND MANAGEMENT IN DOMESTIC ABUSE

> There is a need for a dedicated random sample national survey in the UK. This would estimate more fully the extent and nature of the risks of domestic violence.
>
> (Walby and Myhill 2000: n.p.)

In discussing risk assessment there are a number of important areas to consider, none of which has so far been thoroughly researched in the UK. As domestic abuse is a multi-dimensional occurrence, the client being abused by a current or past partner requires multi-professional, multi-agency intervention. To date there are no comprehensive risk assessment instruments widely available in the UK, although work is currently being undertaken in a number of disciplines. Therefore, healthcare staff need to consult with staff in other areas to provide guidelines for client safety. Taylor-Browne (2001: 111), in a comprehensive literature review, found that a number of authors recommended that health risk assessments should be undertaken on women in abusive relationships. Indeed, Campbell (1986) suggested that the act of undertaking the assessment was sufficient in some circumstances to cause the woman to take positive action. This is hardly surprising, as it is well known that one of the chief survival strategies used by women in abusive relationships is that of denial. Getting a woman to actively engage in assessing the violence might be therapeutic, in which case the activity may well reduce any self-blaming behaviour.

Health risks to clients

Research has demonstrated conclusively that some women who have been abused later present with long-term physical health problems. Therefore, it is crucial that all health assessments recognize this important factor. Staff must recognize that a client who is, or has been, abused might currently be misusing alcohol or drugs. Consequently, this may further compromise their physical and psychological health, which is already being endangered by the partner abuse. Where staff have no readily available assessment instrument, it may be necessary to seek assistance in assessing the mental health status of the client. To ignore this situation could be to jeopardize the client's current and future well-being.

Risk of self-harm

Research has shown that as a last resort some clients in abusive relationships attempt and often succeed in committing suicide. Where the client appears to be depressed or suicidal or in any way mentally dysfunctional, the health professional must consider referral to a member of the mental health team for risk assessment.

Risk to children

The potential harm that can occur to children in an abusive home has already been discussed. Where the health professional has reasons to be concerned, the child health services should be made aware of the situation. Health organizations should have in place comprehensive practice guidelines related to the safety of children in homes where an adult is being abused.

Risk of further abuse

Studies have highlighted factors that may be significant when assessing the likelihood of future domestic abuse, including:

1 *Previous domestic abuse* Studies indicate that a physical assault is rarely a single occurrence in a relationship. Moreover, it is unlikely to exist without accompanying

emotional, psychological and sometimes sexual abuse. In 35 per cent of households a second incident occurs within five weeks of the first (Walby and Myhill 2000: 2).

2 *Time* The most dangerous time for a woman is when she has decided to leave the relationship or soon after she has left. Women who leave an abusive relationship are frequently harassed by their ex-partner after they have left. The British Crime Survey identified 22 per cent of separated women who had been assaulted in the previous year by partners or ex-partners.

3 *Age* Young women between the ages of 16 and 24 are thought to be principally at risk. The research suggests that the violence decreases as a woman gets older (or perhaps she just becomes resigned to the lifestyle and therefore ceases to seek help).

4 *Pregnancy* Evidence indicates that within the 16–24 age group pregnancy adds to the risk factor. International studies have revealed that abuse may begin or escalate with pregnancy.

5 *The relationship* between the couple influences the degree and frequency of the violence. Studies indicate that some men maintain 'traditional' dominant male roles, with some of them believing that it is legitimate to use violence against their female partner. Hearn's study (1996) verified the divergence between men's and women's definitions of violence.

6 *Unemployment* It has been suggested that unemployed women or housewives are more vulnerable to abuse, although some authors contradict this interpretation by presenting the argument that women in high-paid jobs frequently do not report abusive incidents to any authorities.

7 *Poverty* There appears to be a correlation between poverty and domestic abuse although the debate about the 'hidden nature' of domestic abuse in the upper and middle classes may contest these statistics.

8 According to Walby and Myhill (2000) there is supporting evidence that women living in poverty have fewer options, and may therefore be trapped in abusive relationships.

9 *Vulnerable groups* Certain groups are known to be especially vulnerable to on-going abuse due to the fact they may not be able to access outside help. These groups include individuals with disabilities, women from ethnic minorities, particularly if they were not born in the UK and where English is their second language, and others with special needs.

10 According to Mullender (1996) women from ethnic minority groups, and black women, may encounter racism within the institutions from which they are seeking help. This may force them to return to the abusive partner.

(Adapted from Walby and Myhill 2000)

Key point

Research has identified a number of characteristics, which singly or collectively may be indicators of existing or future domestic abuse; nevertheless, there is a convincing argument for further research to identify additional predictors. In the interim health professionals, in collaboration with other agencies and organizations, need to develop risk assessment instruments based on current knowledge. Ideally, elements of client information might be collated and shared between agencies, within the boundaries of confidentiality.

CLINICAL ASSESSMENT OF THE CLIENT WHO HAS BEEN ASSAULTED BY THEIR PARTNER

If a patient has been battered by a partner, the abuse is extremely likely to happen again. In almost all cases, there is nothing the patient can do within the relationship to stop the violence. In many cases, the batterer will apologize and swear to reform. Apologies, however, do not mean that the violence will stop.

(Santa Clara County 1997: 13)

The type of assessment undertaken on a client in an abusive relationship will vary according to the clinical needs of the client, or the health area in which she has presented. The following is a general guide for a health assessment and details that are more explicit will be given when exploring specific healthcare settings.

Key points

Whenever staff have reason to believe the client is being or has been abused by her partner certain principles need to be followed.

The client must always be treated with respect, in a non-judgemental way by all staff. The focus of care must be enabling the clients to make their own choices, in their own time in a manner that preserves their personal safety. The woman should feel empowered to make her own choices.

This may be the first time the client has discussed the abuse with an outsider. When she leaves, she must feel able to seek further help at any point in the future, without fear of recrimination for not taking any previous advice.

Undertaking a general physical examination

Such an assessment may occur routinely if the client presents to her GP or practice nurse with, for example, abdominal pain, chest conditions, or other symptoms, when she has to undress. Staff may notice bruising, abrasions or other signs of physical injury. The district nurse in the course of her daily work may notice a client has unexplained bruising whereas staff in an Accident and Emergency unit more often meet the client when she attends for more serious injuries, or following an incident in which she requires close physical examination. Whatever the circumstances, staff ought to be alert for any of the following.

General demeanour

It is almost impossible to characterize the behaviour or the health need of a woman who is being abused by her partner. For some the injuries are frequent, the psychological abuse constant and the consequences serious and on occasions irreversible. On the other hand, women whose relationship has only recently become abusive may present with little visible evidence that they are being abused. This of course is one reason why routine screening is advised.

What the healthcare professional can do is be on the alert for the following:

- The client may be evasive, or alternatively she may offer an improbable history for any injuries.
- She may make frequent use of health services including the GP surgery, visits to the practice nurse or clinics, often with vague general symptoms with no obvious or easily diagnosed cause.
- Alternatively, the woman may avoid follow-up appointments or routine screening for family planning, cervical screening, breast screening, midwifery care, and post-natal care.
- She may avoid follow-up visits to the health visitor, and the Mother and Baby group, etc.
- She may appear quite apprehensive, particularly if the questions hint around abuse.

Partnership dynamics

Again, it is difficult to attribute specific characteristics to an abusive relationship; indeed, were it easy to spot then arguably fewer women would have to suffer in silence. Interesting studies have been undertaken that attempt to typify both 'victims' and 'abusers'. Whilst such profiles might be worthy of note there is a danger that relying on them causes the professional to miss others who do not fit the profile (Berry 2000: 43), and some experts in the field argue vehemently against such profiling of either the man or the woman. What the health professional needs to remember is that domestic violence can happen to any woman whatever her age, race, creed or social status and that the same can be said for the man who abused her. Nevertheless, it is worth observing for the following:

- The client may be accompanied by her partner and constantly refer to him/her when asked questions.
- Alternatively, the partner may do most of the interacting with the health professional.
- Either or both may minimize any injuries and deny any psychological difficulties the woman may be exhibiting. Abusive men frequently minimize their partners' views, and may well put bruises and other injuries down to her clumsiness.
- The partner may become impatient with the client's behaviour if he feels it is drawing unnecessary attention to them.

Taking a history

A careful history must be taken if staff have any reason to suspect that the client is being abused. In particular staff should observe and note:

- *repeated visits for minor trauma* Some thought needs to be given as to whether records that highlight 'at risk' clients should be kept. For example, in Accident and Emergency departments on-going records are kept of all young children under 5 years of age presenting with accidents. Perhaps similar records need to be kept on other 'at risk' groups.
- *delay in seeking treatment* Studies have shown that either clients may be too afraid to present for treatment or, alternatively, their partners may prevent them from doing so.

- *previous assault* Domestic abuse is, usually, an on-going event rather than a one-off incident requiring medical treatment. Therefore, staff should be on the alert for signs of previous injuries, including old scars, old fractures and bruises.
- *an injury from weapons* (old scars or new signs). The perpetrator may use a variety of implements to inflict physical harm on the client. Studies indicate that women more often use weapons so that if the client is male this may be especially pertinent.

Physical signs of injury

Many of the relevant physical signs have previously been identified in Chapter 2. Where the health professional has reason to be suspicious, it is essential that a member of staff with relevant expertise speak to the client. As the whole process is usually stressful for the client, the fewer people involved with the care the less the woman feels violated.

Charting

According to Bloomington (2001), when domestic violence is suspected, doctors or their designees should make a complete legible record of any acute finding. Location of injuries should be drawn on a body map.

The chart/record should include:

1 the patient's own words, with the use of quotation marks, regarding the causes of the injuries or other important information
2 a description of the patient's injuries: type, extent, age, location
3 any opinion by the healthcare provider as to whether the explanation offered for the injury adequately explains the injury
4 photographs of the patient's injuries if possible
5 past history of physical and sexual abuse
6 documentation regarding maintenance of physical evidence until it has been turned over to police
7 record of referrals.

Individual staff may need to consult their professional body and/or local trust policies for recommendations on confidentiality, disclosure, and legal and ethical implications of detailed record keeping.

Possible interventions

The assessment and management process should incorporate a discussion of the client's *short-term* options and plans including whether she can safely return home. This again depends upon the individual clinical setting and may be most relevant to Accident and Emergency settings where the woman presents with acute physical injury.

In other settings, where the process of leaving may be prolonged, the woman should be advised to make a Personal Safety Plan. Such plans are available from Women's Aid, the local domestic violence forum and occasionally the local police services. Health organizations must ensure that plans are readily available to hand out to clients at risk. A Personal

Safety Plan advises the individual how to plan in advance in case she suddenly has to leave home because the violence has escalated to the point where a rapid exit is her only chance of avoiding serious harm. See Appendix 3 for an example of a safety plan.

Talking to an expert

For those women who are not in immediate danger, or for those who choose not to leave the abusive relationship at that time, it is important that they are encouraged to talk with other agencies. Organizations such as Women's Aid offer on-going advice and support should they need it. As we saw earlier, the most dangerous time for a woman in an abusive relationship, is either at the time she leaves, or soon after she has left.

Many women in abusive relationships may at some point find themselves having to seek refuge either short-term with a friend or family member, or more long-term in one of the refuges across the country. For significant numbers of women it is vital that their destination and new place of residence is kept a secret.

> 'In any one day nearly 7,000 women and children are sheltering from violence in refuges in the United Kingdom' (Women's Aid Federation of England 2001).
> An estimated 19,910 women and 28,520 children stayed in refuges in England in the year ending 31 March 1998. Over 35,000 women called the Women's Aid National Domestic Violence Helpline this year (2000).
> (Women's Aid Federation of England 2001)

If the violence is escalating and the woman fears she may have to leave the house in order to maintain the safety of herself and her children, there are a number of things that she should consider doing in advance, including the following suggestions:

1   Have a spare set of keys made. This should include keys to the house and the car and any other locked areas that she may want to access later.
2   Pack a small suitcase with essential items including changes of clothes, and personal items including valuables that will not be missed by the partner.
3   Pack a small number of children's belongings, but not anything the child is going to miss in the interim and start asking questions about.
4   Where possible, the woman should put important documents in a safe place that can be easily accessed after she leaves. This might include passport, medical certificates, birth and marriage certificates, bank books, post office books, etc.
5   Where possible, the woman is advised to begin to put money aside where it cannot be found by the man. It is imperative that if she opens a secret savings account none of the paperwork is delivered to the house.
6   If any family member is reliant on medication this should be taken when they leave; alternatively it may be necessary to get an urgent prescription the following day.
7   Friends and family must be made to realize the importance of keeping her destination secret. Only those people who absolutely have to know should be told of her whereabouts.
8   Always remember the abused woman is an expert in his anger, she will know better than anyone how potentially dangerous he is. It is important that those around her

respect and support whatever decisions she makes, even if it is supporting her if she returns to the abuser.

The next chapter seeks to explore more specific aspects of assessment according to the client group.

Chapter 6

Domestic violence in a variety of clinical settings

ILLNESS AND INJURY AS A RESULT OF DOMESTIC VIOLENCE

> In addition to injuries sustained during violent episodes, physical and psychological abuse are linked to a number of adverse physical health effects including arthritis, chronic neck or back pain, migraine and other frequent headaches, stammering, problems seeing, sexually transmitted infections, chronic pelvic pain, stomach ulcers, spastic colon, and frequent indigestion, diarrhoea, or constipation.
>
> (Family Violence Prevention Fund 1999 [http://www.fvpf.org])

The short-, medium- and long-term effects of domestic abuse on health were discussed in Chapter 2. This chapter will focus on specific health needs including emergency care, mental health intervention, pregnancy, rape, sexual assault, and aspects related to the health and well-being of children. It explores the role of specialist healthcare groups including staff working in Accident and Emergency settings, GP practice settings, paediatrics, obstetrics and gynaecology, community and other acute care settings.

In all areas of healthcare, staff meet clients who have experienced, or are experiencing, abuse within an intimate relationship. Therefore, staff at every level of an organization ought to have an understanding of domestic abuse and its implications for the clients and the care they require. There should also be other staff with more detailed knowledge relevant to explicit situations such as emergency care, follow-up care or community care.

STAYING SILENT

When discussing or analysing any aspect of domestic abuse it is important to take into account the mounting feminist discourse on the subject which emphasizes the implications of the wider social origins of abuse. Historically, in seeking to explain domestic abuse, research studies have concentrated on the actions or mind-sets of the individual woman (victim) or abuser, or on their interactions with one another. With such a focus, studies then may fail to acknowledge the substantial impact that gender inequalities play in the overall state of affairs.

Whilst it may be informative for practitioners to analyse psychological and social characteristics of the individual, it is equally important to appreciate that to do so without accepting the wider picture minimizes the problems faced by those being abused. Moreover, such a restricted methodology limits the variety of interventions accessible to all concerned. Nevertheless, an exploration of current themes related to domestic abuse in healthcare is essential to an overall understanding of the client's needs, and therefore this chapter explores diverse approaches to the subject.

Research studies routinely confirm that women repeatedly remain silent about abuse for several years before they finally inform someone. Other women remain silent for ever. There are numerous valid explanations offered for the woman's silence, but the most important is that for many women, silence is the only option. Until a wide range of services are available which enable women to seek adequate, independent housing, income, child care, and employment to provide a safe home for themselves and their children, many thousands of women have little choice but to stay put. Moreover, leaving does not guarantee freedom from partner abuse because for countless women the harassment and accompanying violence often continue for months or even years.

Why do women stay silent?

> The cost of maintaining silence is high. When no action is taken, violence in intimate relationships usually escalates. The health and well-being of a woman in such an on-going situation will deteriorate and her use of health services will increase.
>
> (Ingram 1994: 146)

Asking why the woman stays silent is the same as asking why she does not leave, when really the question should be why does he abuse her? Nevertheless, practitioners do need to be aware of the reasons women have given for staying silent, especially when these relate directly to the healthcare they have previously received. A variety of explanations exist as to why a woman (or indeed a man) chooses not to confide in healthcare staff that she or he has been injured by her or his partner, some of which have been covered in previous chapters. However, the following is a summary of what are thought to be the internal and external pressures on women to prolong the silence.

STAYING SILENT

Reasons for staying silent may include:

- *Fear* The woman may be silent out of fear that her partner will discover she has disclosed to someone and will punish her for not maintaining the silence. The shame of what others, including close friends and family, might think may accompany the fear that if others know they may not honour the secret.
- *Mistrust of healthcare professionals* If the woman shares the knowledge of the violence then her safety becomes dependent upon the silence of others, thus increasing her vulnerability. This is particularly relevant if she is afraid for her children, or anxious that they might be taken into care.
- *Shame* Frequently women develop low self-esteem after long periods of abuse. The woman may have been persuaded that the violence is in part, or in total, her own fault. Over time, she may be persuaded that her 'behaviour', her 'lack of skills as a wife and mother', her 'lack of sexual appeal', her 'looks' (these are his claims, not the

reality), etc., have contributed to the violent outbursts. She is perhaps conditioned to believe that no alternatives exist.

- *Lack of resources* The woman is possibly unaware that help from outside agencies is available, and thus is unable to design a plan of alternative action.
- *Lack of support* If a woman has previously sought help and it was not forthcoming then the likelihood of her trying again diminishes. Equally, if previous attempts to support her were directive rather than supportive, and if the advice given was ignored, she may fear going back again. Therefore, it is important for staff to understand that leaving a violent relationship is a process and not a single act, and the key to leaving is often empowerment.
- *Dependency* Abuse in intimate relationships is usually a combination of physical, psychological, emotional, sexual, and financial aspects. Ultimately the woman could be totally reliant upon her partner and devoid of independent resources, so that leaving is not a viable option.
- *Reality* The healthcare professional ought never to underestimate the reality of the woman's assessment of the situation. The knowledge that leaving is not the end, knowing for certain that he will follow her, continue to threaten and possibly even kill her, makes her decision to stay a strategic one of survival.

BATTERED WOMAN'S SYNDROME (BWS): A CRITIQUE

According to the BMA (1999: 31), the battered woman syndrome is a traumatic pathological attachment resulting in an extreme form of co-dependency based on a relationship of fear rather than bonds of affection. The individual experiences a range of frequently debilitating symptoms including acute anxiety, hyper-vigilance, acute and continuous stress responses, periods of extreme sadness and possibly depression, and on occasion feelings of overwhelming helplessness. Over time the woman finds herself emotionally and psychologically 'disabled' with little choice but to stay.

However, several feminist authors challenge the thinking that underpins some current psychological explanations of domestic abuse (Dobash and Dobash 1992; Mullender 1996; Bartal 1998). These and other authors argue that theoretical explanations, including that of post-traumatic stress disorder, and battered wife syndrome, especially when used in a court of law to explain why the woman fought back, are inappropriate. BWS emerged originally in the United States to become a recognized defence for women who seriously assaulted or killed their abusive partner, especially whilst he slept or was incapacitated through alcohol. As a defence it became a viable alternative to a charge such as murder, which carries with it a mandatory life-sentence. Mullender states that:

> there are problems with these labels because they portray passivity and psychological damage rather than justifiable defence, but the current state of the law on murder allows women few options, so lawyers use what they think will be helpful.
>
> (Mullender 1996: 50)

According to authors such as Mullender, using BWS as a defence is essentially blaming the woman for what in reality is an act of self-defence. However, until the law is changed others in the field, such as defence counsel, will continue to use the classification, especially in criminal justice cases.

> BWS emphasizes damaged women, rather than women who perceive themselves to be, and may in fact be, acting competently, assertively and rationally in the light of alternatives. The legal focus becomes trying to find an 'excuse' rather than a justification linked to a reasonable act.
>
> (Justice for Women undated)

Nonetheless, other authors advocate the use of this classification to enhance professionals' understanding of the subject area. In certain circumstances, these models are useful, though it is essential not to discount the fact that theories of individual biological or psychological pathology have restricted application, often because they are based on stereotypical behaviour.

> In cases of battered women who kill their violent partners, it might be possible to argue that fear and despair might also constitute relevant characteristics for the purpose of fulfilling the objective test in provocation defences. Battered woman syndrome is not a psychiatric diagnosis, and therefore will rarely constitute sufficient grounds for a diminished responsibility defence. However, the psychological, behavioural and cognitive deficits encompassed within the syndrome may be important in terms of considering relevant characteristics for the purpose of a Section 2 (provocation) defence.
>
> (Mezey 2001: 544)

Mezey is signifying that whilst BWS may in itself not be a legal defence, the adverse clinical manifestations within the woman as a result of the abuse, can possibly be regarded in a court of law as a reasonable response to provocation.

There are women who present to healthcare settings manifesting the 'symptoms' outlined in BWS, or post-traumatic stress disorder, and therefore professionals ought not to ignore its potential for use in healthcare; rather they should keep an open mind. Additional research is required in this and other spheres; in the meantime, healthcare professionals are required to utilize all the tools at their disposal to comprehend the implications of abuse in intimate relationships.

DOMESTIC ABUSE AND MENTAL HEALTH

> Individuals with unrecognized anxiety, depression, or other problems present themselves more frequently for somatic complaints, undergo multiple, negative organic workups, and receive ineffective, symptomatic treatments.
>
> (American Medical Association 1995b [http://www.ama-assn.org])

It has long been established that domestic abuse and violence can have devastating effects on an individual's mental well-being. This section outlines research previously undertaken in this field, including recent debates around healthcare needs in relation to the mental well-being of domestic violence survivors.

Staff attitudes to clients

Research studies consistently demonstrate that women in established violent and abusive relationships may have long-term alcohol and drugs-related problems. Whilst this may bring them to the attention of healthcare professionals there is no guarantee that their dependency is overtly linked to the violence at home. Indeed, Miller *et al.* (2000: 1290) show that:

> For instance, clinicians and policy-makers in various health care and intervention settings have postulated that victimization may decrease the probability that a woman will seek treatment for alcohol and other drug problems if seeking such treatment increases the negative reactions by the perpetrator.

Size and nature of the problem

Summarizing studies of the mental health needs of women in abusive relationships Gerlock (1999) established that women in abusive relationships, when compared to women who have not been abused, more frequently:

- experience stress-related illnesses
- present with psychosomatic illnesses
- experience periods of depression and anxiety
- have low self-esteem
- visit their physician. (McPherson [1994] discovered that where domestic abuse had been identified, family members visited the physician eight times more often than families in homes where domestic abuse was absent.)

There is insufficient data undertaken into the mental health profile of the abusive males to offer any conclusions. However, in Gerlock's study he identified men known to be abusers, who reported negative health outcomes in both medical and mental health problems:

> Health care providers tend to think of negative health consequences as happening only to victims of DV. Indeed, health injuries and problems related to DV are well documented for victims. When one works with domestically violent men it quickly becomes apparent that they generate self-injuries as well as other physical and mental health consequences as a result of their behaviours.
>
> (Gerlock 1999: 375)

In addition, the American Medical Association (1995b) identifies the following common mental health disorders associated with family violence that can affect any member of the family:

- self-neglect, malnutrition, dehydration; failure-to-thrive in babies
- sleep disorders
- aggression towards self and others
- dissociate states

- repeated self-injury
- eating disorders
- compulsive sexual behaviours, sexual dysfunction
- poor adherence to medical recommendations.

Furthermore, the AMA suggests that any mental health preconditions may be exacerbated in women who are being abused.

> Domestic violence may also aggravate co-morbid psychiatric disorders, and women with psychiatric histories may find their complaints of abuse mistakenly regarded as delusions or other evidence of psychopathology. Women who are immigrants, developmentally or physically disabled, from cultural backgrounds different from the physician, or who do not speak the dominant language are also at higher risk for not having their complaints taken seriously.
>
> (AMA 1995b [http://www.ama-assn.org])

Para-suicide

When undertaking her research Williamson (2000), was astonished to discover the high number of incidents reported by staff who took part in the research, of women who had attempted suicide at least once. She later discovered that comparative studies established that at least one in six abused women attempt suicide at least once, and many try several times (Stark and Flitcraft, 1996: 100). Williamson revealed that research in the field of domestic abuse demonstrates how in some studies, up to 40 per cent of women in refuges have attempted suicide, a figure far greater than women in the wider population. Perhaps not surprisingly, her research supported earlier studies that established how significant numbers of healthcare staff repeatedly viewed the event as a 'cry for help', rather than a serious attempt to end life.

Screening mental health clients

Mezey's study (2001), in which she was establishing the existence and use of screening protocols for domestic violence in several healthcare settings, noticed that: 'Reviewing the notes, the authors found that psychiatric patients or patients with a psychiatric history were significantly less likely to be screened than non-psychiatric patients, even though this group is arguably at particularly high risk' (2001: 546). This occurs despite the fact that it is known that victims of domestic violence have increased rates of depression, anxiety, post-traumatic stress disorder, and alcohol and substance misuse, as a consequence of the violence. Arguably, failure to undertake routine screening or carry out an appropriate risk assessment in mental health areas could be construed as negligence.

POST-TRAUMATIC STRESS DISORDER (PTSD)

Post-traumatic stress disorder, according to the BMA (1999: 31), 'refers to a range of psychological responses in people exposed to traumatic and life-threatening experiences including military combat, natural disasters, terrorist attacks, rape and inter-personal violence'.

PTSD as a healthcare phenomenon emerged as a consequence of doctors seeking explanations for the medium- and long-term negative experiences that soldiers reported long after a war was over. The research was later extended to make sense of the experiences of people who had suffered other life-threatening or life-altering events such as major incidents. Individual responses to a life-threatening event often share similar characteristics which include:

- *numbing:* a feeling of total disbelief that such an event could have occurred. The client may well behave as though nothing has happened if she or he slips into a state of denial. The numbing can become a long-term coping strategy that denies a sense of reality to the person experiencing it.
- *fear:* a sense of fear may lead to the feeling that there is no certainty in anything in her or his life. This is particularly relevant to individuals who have been raped or sexually assaulted by an intimate partner. Most people feel comparatively safe within their own homes and the need to be vigilant at home is not a persistent concern. However, being violated by someone so close leads to a need to re-evaluate one's whole life. Many of the events occur without warning and the individual is left feeling powerless for an indeterminate period.

Other symptoms, which persist for many months, can include:

- intrusive recollections of the assault
- 'waking flashbacks', experienced with an intense sense of reality
- vivid and often terrifying dreams of the assault
- intense psychological and physiological distress, provoked by internal and external cues that remind the client of the attack. A sound, smell or word can trigger an autonomic response that leaves the client feeling powerless.
- physiological over-reactivity, including exaggerated startle response
- avoidance of discussing the attack, pretending it did not happen at all
- avoidance of places, people, or things that recall the attack
- feeling of being apart from other people or that there is no future
- insomnia, irritability, and trouble concentrating.

Key point

Individuals differ regarding their capacity to cope with catastrophic stress so that while some people exposed to traumatic events, including domestic abuse and violence, do not develop PTSD, others go on to experience the full-scale syndrome. Therefore, any psychological assessment needs to acknowledge the resilience of some women to endure high levels of abuse and to develop sophisticated coping strategies.

According to the BMA (1998: 31), studies illustrate that women who have experienced domestic violence are more prone to develop psychiatric illnesses including PTSD, anxiety, and depression, than are women who have not. Williamson (2000) says that professionals in the field, who continue to debate the efficacy of applying labels such as PTSD and BWS, argue that to do so diminishes the significance of the source of violence:

> If a patient is considered in relation to cultural myths and stereotypes, which minimise her experiences of violence and abuse, then it is possible for healthcare professionals to diagnose a woman's psychological symptoms in relation to psychiatric problems which subsequently minimise the role and impact of domestic violence.
>
> (Williamson 2000: 21)

Gondolf (1995: 36) expressed concern that if healthcare professionals fail to consider the psychological symptoms collectively then a misdiagnosis may occur. He believes certain symptoms such as avoidance behaviour, hyper-vigilance and extreme anxiety are by themselves signs of a psychiatric disorder. However, when viewed collectively in a woman who is being abused at home: 'These extremes taken together suggest a person with PTSD with an unpredictable and threatening environment'.

RAPE TRAUMA SYNDROME

> It is now accepted that the experience of rape and serious sexual assault is associated with severe emotional, cognitive and behavioural consequences in a significant proportion of victims.
>
> (Royal College of Psychiatrists 1996: 12)

First described in the 1970s, rape trauma syndrome is now generally acknowledged as a variant of post-traumatic stress disorder (PTSD). According to the Royal College of Psychiatrists in 1996, significant numbers of women who have suffered from sexual assault and rape go on to suffer from long-term problems:

> About one third of women who report rape develop long-term psychological and social problems, including problems in relating at an intimate or trusting level, sexual dysfunction, persisting anger and irritability, helplessness and excessive dependence, loss of confidence and self-esteem.
>
> (Royal College of Psychiatrists 1996: 12)

Following the initial attack a woman or a man, sexually assaulted by their current or ex-partner, may develop signs of rape trauma syndrome. If this occurs she or he should be referred to the appropriate medical and/or voluntary support agencies. Healthcare professionals working in mental health settings are aware of the appropriate clinical interventions for clients requiring care for any of the above. What is essential is for all units to have in place correct and effective procedures for the assessment and management of care, in particular when a client requires multi-agency intervention, or is found to be especially vulnerable.

MENTAL HEALTH SERVICES AND VULNERABLE CHILDREN AND YOUNG PERSONS

> All professionals working in mental health services in the statutory, voluntary and independent sectors, should bear in mind the welfare of children, irrespective of whether they are primarily working with adults or with children and young people.
> (Department of Health [DoH] 1999b: 28, 3.39)

The Department of Health (1999) clearly distinguish the critical role that staff from within mental health services are required to play in relation to child protection issues. Logically therefore, staff ought to be trained in the complex issues surrounding children living within an abusive home, especially those associated with potential adverse mental health consequences. 'They should follow the child protection procedures laid down for their services within their area. Consultation, supervision and training resources should be available and accessible in each service' (Department of Health [DoH] 1999b: 21).

Whatever healthcare setting an abused woman presents to, qualified staff at all levels need appropriate knowledge to recognize what help is required and whom the woman needs to be referred to. This is particularly relevant to clients presenting with mental health needs, as failure to recognize their immediate healthcare deficit could lead to long-term or even fatal consequences. Equally important is the need for healthcare staff to recognize the point at which a client requires mental health intervention rather than counselling or unsupervised drug therapy. Failure to anticipate the specific mental and physical needs of women in abusive relationships might lead to serious ill-health consequences including suicide.

CARE OF CLIENTS IN THE ACUTE CARE SECTOR

Women who are, or have been, abused may present to a mixture of clinical settings, for a variety of reasons, with a range of clinical needs. There are occasions when the visit is not, or does not appear to be, directly related to a condition linked to domestic abuse; however, healthcare professionals ought to be alert for any signs that the woman is being abused. For example, a woman who has been sexually abused by her partner may present with indeterminate clinical needs to a specialist genito-urinary clinic, within a family planning clinic, or within a gynaecological department. A sexually transmitted infection is not an uncommon feature of domestic abuse, but failure by the professional to ask the correct questions, or an assumption that the client is engaging in high-risk sexual encounters willingly, may inhibit disclosure, and thus limit health-intervention options. Equally, practitioners within an orthopaedic setting, including radiology, may receive clients presenting with injuries acquired as a result of physical assaults. Other women utilize the services of ophthalmic specialists, fascio-maxilliary units, medical or surgical units, or they may be admitted to any acute or critical care area.

DOMESTIC VIOLENCE IN ACCIDENT AND EMERGENCY SETTINGS

Women who attend Accident and Emergency departments

Over time, statistics have shown that:

- 1:4 women are victims of domestic violence at some point in their life
- 22 per cent–35 per cent women attending Accident and Emergency departments in the UK were doing so directly as a result of domestic violence (Hadley 1992)
- A study by Stark et al. in 1979, further indicated that 1:5 women who attend Accident and Emergency do so as a direct result of intimate violence, and had on average sought medical attention for injuries at least 11 times previously.
- Intimate violence is the major cause of physical injury for women between the ages of 15 and 44 years (Grisso et al. 1991).
- Ingram (1994) highlighted studies, which indicated that despite this, only 1 per cent–6 per cent of these women are actually diagnosed as suffering from the consequences of intimate violence.
- During one week in 1997, a study of patients with facial injuries attending 163 of the Accident and Emergency departments in the UK, found that 24 per cent of these were caused by assault (the male:female ratio was 79:21) (Hutchison et al. 1998).
- The level of injury resulting from domestic violence is severe: of 218 women presenting at an Australian metropolitan Emergency department with injuries due to domestic violence, 28 per cent required hospital admission and 13 per cent required major medical treatment. Of these women, 40 per cent had previously required medical care for abuse.

(Berios and Grady 1991)

Accident and Emergency care

Domestic violence-related injuries range in severity from comparatively minor cuts and bruises to severe beatings and, for some women, death. It is important for staff to be alert to the prospect of partner violence in order that they can organize a period of time when the woman has an opportunity to talk to staff alone. Co-ordinating this can be quite a challenge as the abusive partner is apt to be vigilant, and therefore reluctant to leave his/her partner unaccompanied.

Physical injuries

Hadley (1992) indicates that in the UK between 25 percent and 30 per cent of women attending an Accident and Emergency department have injuries, or medical conditions related to domestic abuse, although many do not disclose the aetiology. Women present either to their GP or to the Emergency department with physical injuries which are most commonly found on:

- the face, including broken jaw, nose, and teeth, black eyes with an accompanying fractured orbital bone

- the back of the head, including skull fractures and/or signs of coup-contracoup injury
- the neck, including attempted strangulation
- chest, including fractured ribs and fractured sternum
- breasts, genitalia and abdomen
- ruptured spleen.

Staff should consider the following injuries as conceivably resulting from domestic violence:

- perforated ear drums
- detached retina or other eye injuries
- burns and scalds, particularly if the history is inconsistent with the injury
- bizarre injuries, including severe bite marks
- poisoning, or swallowing harmful substances.

In addition, Accident and Emergency staff are involved with abused women and men who present to the department as:

- victims of strangulation
- victims of rape and sexual assault
- para-suicide
- undergoing episodes of disruption in mental health
- gynaecological emergencies including miscarriage
- following substance misuse, including alcohol and drug overdoses.

Attempted strangulation

According to Berry (2000), choking is an injury 'peculiarly common in domestic violence cases, far more so than in stranger assaults'. He considers strangulation should be viewed as an indicator that the man who did it be classified as an extremely dangerous abuser. This fact is supported by the risk assessment tool currently (2003) in use by the Metropolitan Police service, who view strangulation as high-risk behaviour on the part of the perpetrator.

Moreover, a client with a strangulation injury may present at an Accident and Emergency unit with relatively minor swelling and redness. However, over the next thirty-six hours the swelling could increase until an airway obstruction occurs. When undertaking risk assessment to predict risk of future injuries, strangulation is an indicator of high-level risk.

Client assessment

The assessment of injuries or clinical conditions follows normal protocols, with priority being given to those aspects of care that are known to be life-threatening. Special care should be taken to document all injuries or other clinical findings, notes should be comprehensive and due consideration given to the fact that medical and nursing records may subsequently be used as evidence or a criminal offence.

Guidelines produced from the British Association for Accident and Emergency Medicine (1993) remind staff that: 'Domestic violence is a crime like all other violent crimes. It should be prosecuted once reported like all other crimes.' The guidelines continue by reminding staff that the patient's wishes for confidentiality must be respected. However, where the patient is incapable of consent 'the consultant in charge must be consulted whether to release information when a "serious arrestable offence" has occurred'.

According to the BMA (1998: 52), the General Medical Council (GMC) makes it clear that 'Where the disclosure of relevant information between healthcare professionals is clearly required for treatment to which the patient has agreed, the patient's specific agreement is not required.'

Accident and Emergency departments need to agree and publish guidelines for staff that relate to the relationship between reported injuries and police procedures. On the one hand, the client has a right to confidentiality but on the other hand, the professional has a responsibility to act if it is thought the patient may be in a life-threatening situation. Therefore, serious consideration must be given as to the correct procedure to follow if there is significant concern from the staff that the patient's life is under threat. Patients need to know that it is possible to seek assistance from the local domestic violence officer (DVO) or the local domestic violence unit (DVU) without action being taken against the perpetrator. Similarly protocols directly related to child protection issues must be in place and followed to the letter if it is thought that there exists a serious threat of harm to the child.

Attempted suicide

Standard protocols should be followed when a client is admitted to the Accident and Emergency department because of a suicide attempt. Again, it is important that, if staff suspect the client is in an abusive relationship, every effort must be made to speak to her or him without the partner being present. Referral to a mental health service is preferable, as the situation leading up to the self-harming behaviour is unlikely to be resolved simply because of the current injury. On-going follow-up care should be made immediately available, if the client is to find short-term relief from the abusive alliance.

Routine screening in Accident and Emergency departments

As with other clinical areas the debate regarding routine screening has yet to be agreed nationally, although generally the professional bodies are advocating its use. A study undertaken in the north-west of England, by Howe et al. (2002), concluded that, not only did the majority of clients agree with routine screening for violence, a greater number were also in favour of health staff reporting such incidents to the police.

> Conclusions: Patients attending Accident and Emergency departments support routine questioning by doctors and nurses about violence. They also support health professionals routinely informing the police in cases of violence. Further research is required into the outcomes of routine and direct questioning in Accident and Emergency of patients about their exposure to violence.
>
> (Howe et al. 2002)

Whilst this was a relatively small study, and not specific to domestic violence, and undertaken in a single Accident and Emergency department, it is nevertheless worthwhile considering reproducing it in other departments, across the country. Utilizing an evidence-based assessment tool that includes a 'body map' to mark injuries enhances the collection of essential data. Senior staff may be required to later give evidence in court and therefore careful and accurate record keeping is essential. It may be appropriate to undertake a risk assessment especially if there are indications that the patient's mental health is compromised. Ensuring that details of local helping agencies and emergency help-lines are widely visible within the departments indicates to clients that staff within the department take domestic violence seriously. Leaflets should be readily available and it may be advisable for a supply to be kept in the ladies toilet areas to ensure privacy.

Often, local domestic violence forums take responsibility for designing a series of leaflets, which are placed in an information pack for distribution to patients. Obviously, care has to be taken to ensure the woman can carry the materials safely without arousing the suspicion of her partner, which is why some organizations including Women's Aid, provide credit-card-sized information cards that can be secreted in a pocket or handbag.

DOMESTIC VIOLENCE AND SEXUAL ASSAULT.

> Rape is a common crime with a conviction rate of below 10 per cent and sentences as low as 180 hours community service.

As we saw in Chapter 2, sexual assault and rape are not uncommon in abusive and violent intimate relationships. The aftermath of sexual abuse in the short and long term varies, with some women not even acknowledging that what took place was an assault. Likewise, their partner may also deny the reality of the assault, as some men believe having sex whenever they wish is their 'marital right'. This may be particularly relevant to women from certain cultural backgrounds where subservience to the husband is, as we have already seen, 'the norm'. Whilst it should be noted that no culture or religion either advocates or outwardly condones sexual assault against wives, what often happens is that the woman is subjugated to the will of the husband. Moreover in a number of countries women have little if any, legal standing in their own right so that rape in marriage is not admitted nor acknowledged.

A woman who has been sexually abused, assaulted, or raped may present in a range of healthcare settings. She may attend Accident and Emergency requiring immediate trauma care. Alternatively, she may go to the midwife if the assault results in pregnancy; may speak to the health visitor when the latter visits the family routinely; may visit the women's clinic for emergency contraception or routine screening, or the sexual screening clinic; or, eventually, the mental health services. Recent statistics reveal that: 'Rapes committed by a person unknown to the victim ("stranger" rapes) formed only 12 per cent of the sample; those committed by acquaintances or intimates accounted for 45 per cent and 43 per cent of cases respectively' (Harris and Grace 1999: 2). Between 1986 and 1997, the number of women reporting rape increased by over 500 per cent. Yet convictions have remained almost static, meaning that whilst in 1977 one in three women reporting rape saw her rapist convicted, in 1996 less than one in ten did. Arguably, the criminal justice system is currently failing women, not simply those who report rape, but every woman, since the message being sent out is that rape is a low-risk, high-reward activity. Where there are signs of recent sexual activity and the patient/client indicates it was non-consensual, then with the client's consent the police surgeon should be notified.

Serious sexual assault

According to the Rape Crisis Federation (2001):

1 'It is an offence for a person to make an indecent assault on a woman.'
(S14(1) Sexual Offences Act 1956)

Many acts of serious sexual violence against women are categorized as indecent assault rather than rape. This is usually because the event did not involve penetration of the vagina by the penis, e.g. in penetration of the vagina any other object such as a bottle or a ringed hand was used.

2 'Indecent assault on a man is a separate offence.'
(S15(1) Sexual Offences Act 1967)

The maximum penalty for indecent assault on either a woman or a man is 10 years' imprisonment.

How the law defines rape

A man commits rape if:

1 he has unlawful *sexual intercourse* with a person who at the time *does not consent* to it, and
2 at that time *he knows* that the person does not consent to the intercourse
3 or *he is reckless* as to whether the person consents to it.

This definition includes both male and female victims and applies whatever the relationship between the persons involved, including between a man and his wife. A man is defined as a male, aged 14 or over. At the time of writing, rape is defined as the non-consensual penetration of the vagina or anus by a penis, which means that in law it is now possible to rape a male. The Home Office is currently (2003) reviewing sex offences legislation and one of the recommendations made is that oral penetration be included in the definition of rape.

For a successful conviction of rape, the prosecution must prove that:

1 the person did not consent, and
2 the man knew that the person did not consent.

A man, however, can argue that he honestly believed a woman consented. Being reckless means there is an obvious risk that the woman was not consenting and the man ignored the risk. For example, where the woman is heavily intoxicated the man has to be sure that she is in fact capable of giving consent, otherwise he might be tried and convicted of rape.

Future risks

It has been recorded that three out of five victims of domestic rape have made previous reports of domestic violence to police, and that the level of escalation of violence can rise rapidly. Taking this and the close proximity of the perpetrator to the victim into account it must be recognized that the next incident could potentially be a murder.

(Metropolitan Police Services 2001: n.p.)

It is vital that healthcare professionals recognize that domestic violence incidents habitually escalate in degree and frequency over time. Hence, the care and advice given to an individual victimized by her partner should reflect this potential for future harm. Some clients may require support to make a complaint about the violent behaviour to the police, or the healthcare professional may wish to encourage the patient to do so for her or his future safety. Whilst it is acceptable for the professional to emphasize the risk of not reporting the incident they should never apply undue pressure. To do so puts the client in a position of unwillingness to return in the future for fear of being judged by those giving care. Staff need to remember that the patient/client might spend a great deal of her or his life being forced or bullied into submission, often disguised as being 'for their own good', so nothing is achieved by excessive pressure from healthcare staff.

Emergency care of the client who has been raped or sexually assaulted

The usual emergency assessment and management protocols take precedence over anything else. The client is first assessed for airway, breathing, etc., and any emergency clinical interventions initiated. Where possible the client's clothing should be kept in an evidence bag in accordance with departmental policy guidelines.

Key points

It is reasonable to expect that each department have, *in situ*, guidelines that cover the collection of evidence and the relationship with the legal community, including the local police. Departments should consider working with the local police service to write and implement policies related to rape management where the injured patient is unable to be taken to the police 'sympathy suite'. Otherwise, vital evidence may be lost, leading to an unsuccessful prosecution at a future date.

Similarly, guidelines related to confidentiality must be adhered to, with recognition given to the fact that rape and sexual assault are considered a serious criminal offence.

Departments should have in place protocols that relate specifically to managing the care of clients suffering from rape and sexual assault.

Please note that it is exceptionally important for staff to know how to deal with the client's relatives, bearing in mind that in a number of occurrences the client has been assaulted by her or his partner.

At the time of the health consultation, the client may not wish the police or the relatives to know the circumstances of her admission. This must remain the client's decision, with healthcare staff providing sufficient information about the process to allow her to make an informed choice. Any local policies should include the collection of samples, clothing, etc., and, providing the patient agrees, a careful and detailed clinical history must be taken. A staff report should include a description of the event in the patient's own words, taking care to record all injuries, with photographic evidence if that facility is available.

The next priority is to create a safe environment that stabilizes the patient sufficiently to:

- obtain informed consent. Where the client has impaired consciousness this may not be possible. In such circumstances the department needs to have in place, guiding principles related to the inter-departmental role of the police services.
- gather the necessary medical and sexual history. It is recommended that notes taken should be quite precise, and written in her/his own words. For example 'the patient stated that her partner hit her in the face twice and then forced her to have intercourse', etc. Any examination should include in-depth descriptions of any and all injuries.
- begin a physical and evidence examination. This of course is dependent upon the severity of the injuries. Where possible, if the need is medically non-urgent, it may be undertaken by a specialist forensic medical officer (FMO) if the DNA evidence, including sperm samples, is to be used in court. The patient should be reassured that even if the evidence is collected she can later withdraw the complaint if she so wishes.

The American Medical Association guidelines and those of the British Association of Accident and Emergency Medicine emphasize the need for healthcare practitioners to take exceptional care to maintain the psychological integrity of the client. In circumstances where the client has no urgent clinical needs, it may be more appropriate for her or him to be taken to the 'soft suite' or 'sympathy suite' at the local police station. Alternatively, the police service has a national network of forensic medical officers (FMOs), specially trained in the care of individuals who have suffered rape and sexual assault; an FMO could attend the Accident and Emergency department (or other healthcare department) to undertake the examination.

The client has already been severely traumatized; the ensuing process therefore should not leave her (or him) feeling even more violated. This can be achieved by ensuring that:

- the area in which the examination takes place is quiet, and that staff are not repeatedly entering or leaving the space
- the number of staff involved in the care is kept to a minimum
- where possible the client has a choice as to the gender of those caring for her or him

- the client is fully informed of all procedures
- where possible the client controls the pace of the examination
- unnecessary questions should not be asked as this can be detrimental to the client's well-being and may have an impact on future evidence
- where possible the partner should be excluded from the examination area unless the client expressly asks for him or her
- care should also be taken when admitting friends and family without the express permission of the client, as they may put undue pressure on her or him not to disclose too many details
- clients with strong ethnic or religious views on sexuality may require additional support, especially if they do not speak English. For example, exposing their bodies to strangers, especially men, is forbidden in some cultures.

It is inappropriate for the client to be repeatedly asked to describe events. Therefore questioning should be kept to a minimum and undertaken by staff with experience, one reason why utilizing the skills of the FMO may be the preferred option. Each Accident and Emergency unit should have in place protocols for the assessment and management of clients who have been sexually assaulted. Similarly, the department should stock standard kits used for the examination of clients who have experienced a sexual assault. It is recommended that unless the patient requires immediate emergency care the examination and collection of evidence should be undertaken by a qualified forensic medical examiner.

In addition to undergoing a standard trauma examination, and with care, the client is questioned about the specifics of the incident. Questions try to determine what happened and when; the events as they occurred; whether there was vaginal and/or anal penetration; whether the penetration was by a penis and/or other objects; and whether there was forced oral sex. For this reason, the client should be asked not to drink, or take a mouthwash, until swabs have been taken.

- Where possible the history should include whether or not the perpetrator used a condom, and whether he is known to have any sexually transmitted diseases, or supports a high-risk sexual lifestyle.
- A detailed account of injuries is recorded, and where appropriate photographs are taken and any other relevant information is noted (where doubt exists as to relevance the information is automatically recorded). The use of body maps has been found extremely useful for noting injuries with accuracy.
- Vaginal, nasal and oral swabs are taken.

The medical implications for the victim do not cease once the immediate injuries are dealt with. Female clients may have become fertilized during the rape and are therefore faced with the dilemma of whether or not to take the emergency contraceptive pill. Women and men are both advised to undergo testing for sexually transmitted diseases, including periodic blood tests for the presence of the HIV virus.

As another form of control, some men who abuse their partners may engage in high-risk sexual behaviours, including having unprotected sex with multiple partners. Therefore, the woman (or the male client) is advised to undergo these tests if the forced sex was unprotected. Moreover, she has to make a decision about her immediate circumstances including whether or not to report the incident to the police, and whether to return home. If she was assaulted by an ex-partner then possibly she can return home; however, unless and until he is arrested, she remains in danger of further attacks.

The research confirms that women who are sexually assaulted by a current or past partner commonly have significant problems overcoming the psychological and emotional aftermath due to trust violation. Specifically, they have to deal with the certainty that his violence is unlikely to stop unless legal sanctions are employed, whilst accepting that this is a difficult, and sometimes an impossible, choice for them to make. Moreover, escalation in the frequency and severity of the violence is to be anticipated and further sexual assaults may occur (MPS 2001).

A woman living in an ethnic community or with particular religious beliefs may have to endure the additional pressure exerted on her by the family or others in the community not to report the incident to the police. Black and Asian women, and women from other ethnic minority groups, may be aware of, or have previously experienced, racist attitudes from health or police services, thus making it more difficult for them to report the assault. Healthcare professionals must therefore endeavour to extend their understanding of the cultural or religious realities surrounding marital relationships, sexual conduct within those relationships and the pressures the woman may be placed under. Any care is offered in a non-judgemental way giving due respect to the woman's beliefs and wishes.

Longer-term effects

The aftermath of the assault does not cease when the violence stops; for those clients who do appear in court the trauma may be re-lived during and after the trial.

> The rape victim often experiences the court proceedings as a form of secondary victimisation which leaves them feeling humiliated, fearful, angry and deeply disillusioned with the criminal justice system, particularly if she believes that her assailant is wrongly acquitted.
>
> (Royal College of Psychiatrists 1996)

What is more, statistics confirm that a successful prosecution of rape between two people who are in, or have been in, an intimate relationship is much less common than it is in 'stranger rape' cases. The trauma of going through a trial, the feelings of shame and degradation she may be suffering, and the fear of what might happen if he is not convicted may influence the woman not to press charges. Often individuals who experience rape and sexual assault suffer substantial psychological trauma, which may take many weeks, months and for some even years to resolve. Several women (or men) can experience the symptoms of rape trauma syndrome, which is covered in more detail later in this chapter.

Male rape victims

> The legal definition of rape was also altered in 1994, to include penile penetration of the anus. Thus, the offence of male rape has only been part of the criminal law for a short period of time, despite being recognized in the academic literature for some years.
>
> (Home Office 2002)

It is important to recognize that whilst statistics are limited, male rape does occur within intimate relationships, as well as from strangers. When male rape occurs within an intimate relationship, it may be assumed that both men are homosexual. However, it is equally important that in any other incidents of male sexual assault, healthcare staff and staff from other agencies do not assume that the client is homosexual.

Gay or bisexual men reporting rape and sexual assault have the additional trauma of accessing help from individuals within the healthcare services and police services who may be homophobic. Individuals who are transgender have particular issues related to their sexuality, and many professionals are ignorant of the intricacies of this sexual orientation. Repeatedly, staff within such institutions have limited understanding of the health needs of individuals in abusive relationships, clients who have been raped or individuals in gay, bisexual or transgender relationships. Therefore, the experience of a non-heterosexual man in an intimate relationship, who has been raped by his partner, could be extremely challenging. Healthcare staff should address the needs of this minority client group by ensuring staff at all levels have a greater understanding of their needs. Moreover, all employers have a responsibility to ensure that staff within the organization operate in an anti-oppressive, anti-discriminatory manner at all times and that appropriate on-going staff development is available to support this philosophy.

Procedures for dealing with male rape victims are similar to those described above for the care of women who have been raped and contact numbers of organizations can be found in Appendix 1. It should be noted that when a man is raped or sexually assaulted by an unknown male he faces issues significantly different from those facing female victims. Whereas some women may believe they were attacked because of their femininity, men may be left questioning their own sexuality. They may fear that in some way their manner might have given off the wrong message, especially if the attacker(s) were able to cause them to ejaculate. The long-term effects can be devastating and there are few support systems for survivors of male rape, and those that do exist are normally linked to help lines for gay men. The man also needs to undergo tests for sexually transmitted diseases, particularly screening for the HIV virus.

Continuing healthcare needs of clients in sexually abusive relationships

Sexual assault and rape is rarely if ever about sexual gratification, it is about a man exerting ultimate power over the other person, who is usually, although not always, a woman. The abusing partner in an intimate relationship may resort to sexual humiliation and violence to control his partner. He may indulge in potentially hazardous sexual activities outside of the partnership in order to humiliate his partner and may later demand unprotected sex with her or him. He may insist on his partner engaging in sexual activities with other men or sexually abuse her in their presence. Personal accounts of sexual abuse within intimate relationships suggest that even if he knows he is HIV positive, or carrying another sexually transmitted disease, he may insist on unprotected sex.

Domestic abuse and sexually transmitted diseases

An American study into sexually transmitted diseases (STDs) in 2000, using a questionnaire, estimated the percentage of women attendees at a clinic who had experienced domestic violence incidents during their recent relationships. There were 375 female clinic attendees who completed the questionnaire. Of these, 141 (37.6 per cent) women reported having at some time experienced physical assault by an intimate and 123 (32.8 per cent) reported verbal threats of violence. According to 58 (15.5 per cent) of the women there had been at least one episode of physical abuse in the year preceding participation. A report of physical violence was associated with drug use, STD history, and a history of a serious medical condition. Whilst it was recognized that the study was undertaken in a poor inner city area, nevertheless the researchers concluded that STD clinics are an important healthcare site for the detection of abuse and for possible intervention when women are being abused. The recommendation made was that staff in this speciality should be appropriately trained in the various aspects of domestic abuse in order that they might offer suitable care for their clients.

The specific role of the healthcare professionals is to support the client psychologically and emotionally during the assessment and management process.

Again, it is essential that healthcare professionals possess adequate information about the subject if they are to respond in a way that is supportive, empowering and effective. Staff should know where to refer the patient for clinical assessment, and of organizations that offer support for this client group. Departments, community units, etc., should have established protocols for managing clients requiring screening and treatment for STDs, especially where, and to whom, the client can be referred immediately. Specific clinical settings, including Obstetrics and Gynaecology, genito-urinary clinics, and women's clinics should have more detailed and specific protocols and guidelines related to the screening process.

According to the Clinical Effectiveness Group (the Association of Genito-urinary Medicine and the Medical Society for the Study of Venereal Diseases) the presence of a sexually transmitted infection (STI) after sexual assault is likely to have minimal effect on criminal procedures as the patient would be unlikely to prove that the infection did not exist prior to the assualt. The most common STIs found in women who claim to have been sexually assaulted are gonorrhoea, chlamydia and trichomoniasis. In between 50 per cent and 60 per cent of cases the assailant is known to the woman. The Clinical Effectiveness Group identifies the need for all staff to have specific training within this area, and for clinics to establish and maintain relevant statutory, voluntary and other related agencies. In this way the service offered to individuals who have been sexually assaulted will be comprehensive and supportive.

THE PRIMARY HEALTHCARE TEAM

Members of the Primary Health Care Team are in a unique position to empower women who are experiencing violence from known men. It is safe to argue that GPs and healthcare professionals could play a large role in enabling women to see that they are not to blame, empowering women, helping them to recognize that their safety is of importance and giving them information on services.

(Abbott and Williamson 1999: 89)

The role of members of the primary healthcare teams has changed significantly over the last few years, with staff requiring greater skills and the ability to practise in an ever widening degree of specialist knowledge. Research indicates that staff in primary care have a crucial role to play in the recognition and management of the health and well-being of clients, including children, living within abusive relationships.

DOMESTIC VIOLENCE IN GENERAL PRACTICE

When women seek help from statutory agencies, the GP is likely to be high up on the list of those approached. However, the number of women seeking help from their GP's is not clear, and the helpfulness of the GP's is variable.

(British Medical Association [BMA] 1998: 39)

The role of the general practitioner (GP) in the recognition of domestic abuse is a significant one. The GP is well placed to identify acute episodes of abuse, for example, when undertaking clinical examinations; long-term effects of abuse, in patients presenting with somatic illnesses; women presenting with sexually transmitted diseases, and those who are pregnant. As we have seen the benefits of routine screening for violence are disputed, but targeted questioning is not, providing the follow-up support services are in place. There would appear to be little point in persuading a client to disclose abuse if the health providers are then in a position to offer little more than sympathy. Therefore, it is essential that staff within a general practice setting are trained to recognize the existence of domestic abuse and have a fundamental grasp of appropriate interventions. This may range from clinical referrals for specific conditions – for example, fascio-maxillary care, mental health support – to referral to the women's refuge, etc. Each surgery should provide information packs, easily accessible to those visiting it, and visible posters with the telephone numbers of local support services. It may even be appropriate to occasionally run a local domestic violence and abuse awareness campaign over an extended period, and where appropriate focusing on the needs of the specific local communities.

Unfortunately, research indicates that GPs are generally not as pro-active as they might be in the sphere of screening for, or recognizing, abuse, and may not have the appropriate knowledge and skills to offer effective solutions. The BMA (1998) signifies that national and international studies recognize that the limitation of clinical intervention by this group of practitioners is often due to a lack of understanding of the nature of the problem. In addition, historically, as with many other professional groups, domestic violence has been viewed by doctors as a 'family matter', one that has little relevance to their practice. Where interventions have been acknowledged as good practice, they have almost certainly been developed along the medical model of care. According to the BMA, the most common reasons given in a major Canadian study for non-intervention in cases of domestic violence and abuse by family doctors include:

- that it is a private matter
- infrequent patient visits
- unresponsiveness of the patient to questions
- no patient initiative
- no time
- lack of, or inadequate, training

- unresponsiveness of patient to referrals
- that the doctors forgot to ask.

In a recent study undertaken in Ireland, of the 651 women who had experienced one or more violent incidents and later attended the GP surgery, only 78 (12 per cent) reported that their doctor had asked about a partner threatening them. Although the research demonstrated high levels of physical violence, it also showed that only 32 per cent reported it to their doctor, and only four per cent had been asked by their general practitioner if they had been hit, injured or abused by a partner (Bradley *et al.* 2000). Furthermore, the study revealed that the number of women disclosing their experience of domestic abuse was twice as high as those from previous random surveys undertaken in Ireland, an alarming reality.

> For general practitioners and doctors in accident and emergency, asking women about fear of their partner and controlling behaviours may be an acceptable and effective way of identifying those who are experiencing domestic violence. Further qualitative research is needed to examine and develop this strategy.
>
> (Bradley *et al.* 2000: 271)

One of the main findings of the study was that 'Fear of partner and experiencing controlling behaviour were significantly associated with domestic violence'. They also reported that they found anxiety more strongly associated with domestic violence than depression. Furthermore, 77 per cent of all women who responded stated that they were in favour of routine questioning by their usual general practitioner about the issue of domestic abuse. Nevertheless, it necessitates recognition that before routine screening can be implemented, staff require appropriate training in both content and technique. Moreover, sufficient and appropriate literature should be available for both staff and patients/clients; otherwise screening is a futile and potentially damaging exercise.

In 2000, on behalf of the Royal College of General Practitioners (RCGP), Dr Iona Heath in collaboration with Professor Gene Feder, and Dr Jo Richardson compiled a set of guidelines for GPs to inform and guide their practice. The guide also offers a comprehensive reference list for those wishing to explore the issues in more detail. The guidelines are reproduced in Appendix 6 with permission. Similar to other professional bodies, the RCGP has identified key areas that include the defining of domestic violence, including the size and nature of the problem; the guide then offers advice on the following:

- Consider the possibility – understand how to recognize domestic abuse and how to deal with it.
- Emphasize confidentiality – a client needs to feel safe to disclose the circumstances of her abusive home life without fear of unwanted external intervention.
- Ask the question – often the abused client/patient is hoping that someone will ask about the abuse.
- Ensure the documentation is a complete and confidential record.
- Photographic evidence can be very powerful if used by the authorities should the client decide to inform the police services.
- Assess the present situation – what can and should be done to keep the client/patient and their family safe.

- Provide information – a set of leaflets with essential contact numbers on is invaluable for both the client/patient and the other healthcare staff.
- Devise a safety plan – leaving a violent relationship can be an extremely dangerous time; a planned escape is often the safer of a number of options.

Unfortunately, there is a lack of emphasis on the important role of multi-agency, multi-professional co-operation and collaboration. This omission is arguably one that permeates many of the professional guidelines which is perhaps why various reports have commented on the absence of healthcare professionals on many local domestic violence forums.

COMMUNITY PRACTITIONERS

> We believe that all acute and primary care organizations need to develop policies and procedures for responding to domestic violence. Evaluation of these programmes and robust research on interventions based in health services is a priority.
> (Gene Feder, Professor of Primary Care Research and Development, Barts, and Queen Mary's School of Medicine and Dentistry, London, 2001)

The term 'community practitioner' is used to denote any healthcare practitioner who works primarily in the community. Included are district nurses, health visitors, school nurses, practice nurses, occupational health staff, healthcare assistants, dentists and other dental staff, community psychiatric teams, and child protection teams.

The role of the community practitioner

According to Peckover *et al.* (2001: 106) the community practitioner has a vital role to play in the detection, prevention and management of domestic violence in the community. They recognize that primary care trusts (PCTs) have 'responsibility and account-ability for ensuring that high quality healthcare provision is provided and that health outcome targets are met'. It is their suggestion that domestic violence, having been designated a major public health concern, might in fact be identified by PCTs and acute trusts as a health improvement programme. In addition, community practitioners might consider undertaking further evaluation and research of current and future provision in this area.

Home visiting

Arguably, community practitioners, especially community nurses, and healthcare assis-tants are in a position to recognize the partnership dynamics of the couple as they may see them within their home environment. In particular they may be in a position to view first-hand the non-physical abuse such as controlling behaviour, financial abuse, with-holding care, bullying and emotional abuse, especially behaviour that is destructive to the client's self-esteem.

However, asking about the violence may be difficult if the partner is always there for the home visit, ensuring that the woman cannot confide in the visitor. This is particularly challenging if the woman is confined to the house for a long period or indefinitely, as dependency for her care needs may become a weapon used by her partner to ensure compliance. Even if the community practitioner identifies abuse, the woman may be reluctant to take action, leaving the practitioner feeling powerless to act.

The other issue for community practitioners must be the giving of due regard to their own personal safety. Whilst there may be little if any evidence that they are at special risk from abusive partners, nevertheless precautions should be taken. Community services like those in the acute sector require pro-active responses to what has been designated a major public health issue. It is crucial that each service establishes effective policies, protocols and guidelines that staff across the area can follow. Policies based on recognized good practice enable the community team and the individual practitioner to deal with domestic violence in an informed, safe and practical manner. As the demarcation lines between community health services and social services gradually diminish and the teams move closer to a multi-professional, multi-agency co-operation, the service made available to abused women should improve.

Health visitors

It felt as if domestic violence was a 'private' feature of health-visiting work and not a public issue on the professional agenda. This appeared to influence the extent to which individual health visitors had taken domestic violence on board as a practice issue.

(Peckover 1998: 408)

Peckover's study of health visiting in 1998 indicated that generally there appeared to be a lack of sufficient knowledge, understanding and awareness of many of the health issues related to women in abusive relationships. The study, although small, identified that dealing with families where domestic abuse was prevalent was a significant part of the average health visitor's workload, but few had been offered the opportunity to undertake formal education and training in this area. Equally, the study indicated that all too often health visitors lacked appropriate support when dealing with families experiencing domestic violence. Generally, the female clients interviewed experienced difficulties in talking to health visitors about domestic violence, and felt that the information and support offered were limited. Such findings are perhaps unsurprising as the results reflect several studies undertaken at that time in a multiplicity of other healthcare settings. The fact that the Community Practitioners and Health Visiting Association (CPHVA) has recently produced a comprehensive training pack for practitioners and teachers, signifies a major change in perception of the importance of addressing domestic violence in community settings.

Key points

The current role of the health visitor, including their responsibilities in relation to domestic violence, has been clearly defined in the Department of Health publication in 2001 *The Health Visitor and School Nurse Development Programme.*

What can health visitors do?

- The safety of the woman (and any dependent children) is the paramount consideration in work in this area.
- Listen, establish empathy and trust.
- Empower people to make informed decisions and choices about their lives, and do not try to make decisions on their behalf.
- Respect confidentiality and privacy, and recognize the potential dangers if these are breached.
- Provide regular support to women's refuges and their residents.
- Work closely with other agencies.
- Ensure that you do not place yourself or your colleagues in a potentially violent situation.
- Lobby for local services that are responsive to family needs, for example, anger management sessions.
- Work with other agencies to ensure consistency of approach.

Checklist

- Respect and validation: when a client makes a disclosure, it is essential that your response is sympathetic, supportive, non-judgemental and confidential.
- Response and risk assessment: an immediate response should be made to physical injuries and the client be referred for assessment and treatment.
- Counselling may be necessary. You should undertake an assessment of safety.
- Record keeping: take extreme care when documenting domestic violence. Any record of domestic violence should be kept separately from other notes to maintain confidentiality.
- Information giving: people who are victims of violence should be given information about where they can go for help. You could make contact with other agencies on behalf of the person and, if appropriate, children.
- Support and follow-up: continuity of care is very important in building trust. This also allows you to monitor the situation and check for signs of escalating violence and increasing risk.

    (From the Department of Health, *Health Visitor and School Nurse Development Programme* (2001: 65), used with permission of the Department of Health)

Dentists

A common type of injury sustained by women in abusive relationships includes fascio-maxilliary injuries, fractured orbital bone, jaws (mandibles), and noses. Whilst the history of these injuries might be quite difficult to hide, broken teeth are more easily camouflaged as accidental. Therefore, it is reasonable to expect dentists and dental nurses to have an awareness of domestic violence and to provide support and advice where necessary.

DOMESTIC VIOLENCE IN PREGNANCY

Conclusive evidence has demonstrated that pregnancy, far from being a time of peace and safety, may trigger or exacerbate male violence in the home. Where abuse is suspected, it is the midwife's duty to question the woman involved explicitly but carefully.

(Royal College of Midwives 1997)

Numerous studies indicate that physical violence inflicted by a partner, either may begin in pregnancy or be exacerbated during it. However, the psychological and emotional abuse may have existed for some time. The evidence suggests that the post-partum period is the most dangerous time for the woman and her child.

Key point

The possible health risks to mother and child include an increased risk of:

- miscarriage
- low birth rate
- premature birth
- chorioamnionitis
- foetal injury
- foetal death – still birth

Other factors include:

- The pattern of assault to the pregnant woman may alter, and she is potentially at high risk of multiple-site injuries and to be struck in the abdomen and breasts.
- Studies indicate that the risk of moderate to severe violence is greatest in the post-partum period.
- The foetus may be indirectly harmed if the mother is prevented from seeking medical assistance when injured.
- Increased drug and alcohol use, smoking and suicide attempts in abused women who are pregnant are all potentially injurious to the developing foetus.

continued

In addition Mezey *et al.* (2001) found that women who reported violence during their pregnancy and over the previous 12 months frequently complained of:

- backaches
- headaches
- hyperemesis during pregnancy
- false labour
- minor ailments, abdominal pain, joint pains, etc.
- frequency in passing urine

'Up to 25 per cent of women seen at ante-natal clinics may have experienced severe physical, emotional or sexual abuse' (Abbassi 1998). According to the BMA (1998: 58) in 1997, the Royal College of Obstetricians and Gynaecologists (RCOG) published guidelines for staff related to the need for confidentiality in cases where violence is an issue. In addition, they recommended that staff should undertake training in all aspects of domestic violence in order that they can offer an improved service to abused women.

In December 1997, the Royal College of Midwives (RCM) published a position paper on domestic violence, and its impact on maternal and infant health outcomes. The RCM has advised midwives that ignoring domestic violence as a potential and actual health hazard to both the mother and the foetus is no longer an option. For the first time, in 1999, the report on confidential enquiries into maternal deaths (Department of Health [DoH] 1998) identified maternal death caused by violence from an intimate partner to be a recordable cause of death. In addition, the RCM guidelines state that all midwives should be aware of the services and resources available locally in order that they can offer women a range of options, including referral to another agency, should a woman disclose that she is in an abusive relationship. In addition, in the future the RCM should work with other professionals and voluntary agencies to develop and promote a multi-disciplinary approach to care and support. The document also offers advice on how to engage with routine screening programmes in order that practitioners can improve their assessment skills.

A major study undertaken by Mezey *et al.* (2001) uncovered some disturbing facts about domestic violence during pregnancy:

> Having any history of domestic violence was significantly associated with unemployment (woman and partner); the woman being single, separated or divorced; smoking and illicit drug use; social problems and/or special needs; history of psychiatric illness; history of gynaecological problems; younger age at first pregnancy; and having more previous pregnancies.

However, whether this might have been in some way connected to the locality in which the data was collected has not yet been determined.

Recognizing domestic abuse

In addition to the above signs, the medical and midwifery staff should be alert to the following key point.

Key point

Additional problems for the mother during and/or after pregnancy may include:

- an unplanned pregnancy with gynaecological problems, including sexually trans-mitted diseases
- postnatally some women have presented after forced removal of perineal sutures
- acute or chronic stress, which may lead to disturbed sleep patterns, not eating, or over-eating, inadequate self-caring
- acute anxiety, including hypervigilance, anxiety attacks, stress behaviour patterns
- clinical depression which may lead to self-harming behaviour
- inability to cope with pregnancy which may subsequently lead to inability to cope with the new-born baby
- frequent need for prescribed tranquillizers

Staff issues

The issues for the medical and midwifery staff are similar to those across the range of healthcare settings. In addition, staff need to acknowledge that the new baby and any other children are potentially in a dangerous home environment. Therefore, maternity units and community maternity services should establish clear guidelines for staff on how to deal with any immediate issues including confidentiality, as the life of the mother and/or baby may be in danger, as might the lives of existing children. It is essential that staff work with other professional and voluntary bodies to ensure their safety.

It is suggested by the Royal College of Obstetricians and Gynaecologists in their report 'Violence against Women', that: 'In order to facilitate disclosure of sensitive information, all pregnant women should have one consultation with the lead professional involved in her pregnancy care which is not attended by the partner or by any family member'. Specific issues for staff in maternity services includes record keeping. Pregnant mothers often keep their medical records including their birth plans for the duration of the preg-nancy, designed to ensure continuity in care. However, it does mean that were the preg-nant woman to divulge any information regarding partner abuse or violence he (or she) would have easy access to those records. In addition, for some time it has been recognized as good practice that both parents are encouraged to attend at pre- and post-natal classes and to be actively engaged in the birthing process. Whilst this may be considered the 'ideal' for many women, for those who are being abused it means it is extremely difficult to talk to the midwife or obstetrician without their partner being present. Indeed an abusive partner often goes to great lengths to ensure she is not left alone with a staff member. He may be the first to explain any injuries or bruises, often blaming them on the woman's stupidity, clumsiness or lack of self-caring ability. 'Rather than ignoring the issue, midwives, general practitioners, and obstetricians must develop clinical practices that recognize the risk and enhance the safety of women and their unborn children' (Mezey and Bewley 1997).

The RCM and the RSOG have individually explored the possibility of advocating for at least one ante-natal visit to be for the woman alone. Then she can discuss any fears she may have, and it offers the professional an ideal opportunity to explore issues related to abuse. Similarly, both professional bodies have cautiously recommended that maternity staff explore the potential for routine screening during pregnancy. Significantly, both have made the recommendation that staff should attend training and development events, and they agree categorically that it is appropriate to have in place recognized and effective protocols and procedures related to various aspects of domestic abuse.

In a study undertaken by Marchant et al. in 2001, 183 (86 per cent) of the 211 NHS trusts providing maternity care participated in the survey. It was found that 12 per cent of units had written policies for identifying women experiencing domestic violence, and a further 30 per cent had some form of agreed practice. However, it was established that less than half the maternity units routinely offered women an appointment without their partner, and only just over half displayed material about domestic violence in places where women receive maternity care. At the time of the study, only three units had undertaken audits on their domestic violence practices. They concluded that:

> It is evident that clear guidelines for identification and referral, training, audit and the integration of domestic violence policies with child protection and other policies are necessary to fully address the issues.
>
> (Marchant et al. 2001: 165)

Thus, it can be seen that obstetricians and midwifery staff have an important role to play in the assessment, recognition and intervention in the care of pregnant women living with an abusive partner. Departments need to collectively agree protocols related to awareness raising of staff and clients, routine screening during pregnancy, and possible referral to the health visitor if concerns related to children manifest themselves. For a more pro-active response, establish a collaborative working group with other departments and agencies enabling the obstetric and midwifery team to create a safe environment where staff are well trained in the subject of domestic abuse. This approach engenders a mutual understanding that enhances the care of the woman and her child.

The chapter has verified that health professionals in all settings meet women in abusive relationships, and that any accompanying children may also be at risk. The various professional bodies have begun to address the issues of domestic abuse with many making firm statements about the required elements of 'good' practice. The next step is for all healthcare staff to recognize that an urgent need to develop evidence-based practice across the whole range of healthcare settings, exists as a matter of priority.

Chapter 7

Domestic violence and children

> There is evidence of co-occurrence of domestic violence and child abuse within the same family. Child abuse can be seen as an indicator of domestic violence in the family and vice versa.
>
> (Walby and Myhill 2000: 2)

NATURE OF THE PROBLEM

Not surprisingly, there is an increasing acceptance that a compelling correlation between domestic violence and child abuse exists. Hague and Malos (1998: 19) argue that living in a home where violence against a parent is the norm is in itself abusive to the child. Arguably, this strengthens the debate as to whether or not we should be moving away from the term 'violence' and towards that of 'abuse'; recognizing that physical, psychological, social, financial and emotional abuse are often collective elements of a violent and abusive relationship. Simply focusing on physical acts may result in countless individuals and families continuing to co-exist in homes where abuse, and thus fear, is the norm. This was highlighted by Humphreys (2000), who, in a retrospective analysis of families with a history of violence, discovered that social work intervention either avoided or minimized the issues of domestic violence, or they took a confrontational approach, which often led to removal of the children from the home.

CHILDREN AT RISK

The 1996 BCS statistics revealed that half of those women who experienced partner violence in the previous year were living with children under 16, and 29 per cent reported that the children had been aware of what was happening. Where women suffered recurring violence, at least 45 per cent reported that their children had been aware of the latest incident. In all probability children are affected by 'fear, distress, and disruption to their lives' resulting in significant, adverse, long-term effects depending upon 'their developmental stage, personality and individual circumstances'. Children persistently experience a variety of emotions including fear, powerlessness, and intimidation (Mullender 2000: 1). However, Mullender argues persuasively that in viewing children as victims we may make the mistake of perceiving them to be passive bystanders, whilst many develop sophisticated coping strategies. In contrast, there are notable accounts of how children take on the role of rescuer, phoning for help when their mother is being beaten, giving evidence against the man in court or even physically intervening between the parents whilst the abuse is occurring (Mullender 1996: 152).

It is essential that healthcare practitioners remember that 'Children experiencing domestic violence are exposed to a variety of abusive behaviours and it is crucial that the focus both in research and in practice does not become too narrow in favour of physical abuse, particularly extreme physical violence' (McGee 2000a: 79).

Key points

In a qualitative study on the effects of domestic violence on children, McGee's (2000b) study, along with other research, revealed that:

- Children do not have to suffer physical violence to experience long-term negative effects of living in a home where extreme controlling behaviour and abuse are, or become, the norm. Holden and Ritchie (1991), not surprisingly, did find that children more often experienced negative fathering from the domestic violence perpetrator than did other children.
- In order to maintain their own safety, children may choose, or be forced, to take the father's side in an argument, and may themselves be abusive to their mother (Kelly 1996).
- Often the children live in a very controlled environment in which one small misdemeanour leads to a violent response from the abusing parent (or partner of the mother).
- Children may experience considerable dissonance as they try to comprehend and deal with the dynamics of the situation.
- Children regularly experience a sense of total powerlessness, wishing they could assist their mother, which may produce harm to their long-term emotional well-being.
- This may later cause revenge fantasies, but at the time often leads them to have an overpowering need to stay in the room.
- The child or adolescent may themselves be threatened by the abusive partner with what might happen to them at some future date.
- It is not unusual for the child or young person to blame themselves for what is happening to their mother, particularly as the partner may have used their behaviour as a reason for losing his temper.
- Young people sometimes fear social services will remove them from the home if it is known violence and abuse exists. (The partner may also use social services as a threat to ensure obedience from the mother.)
- Gaudoin (2001: 27) provided evidence confirming that two-thirds of the residents in refuges are children.
- If there is no proof of direct child abuse and the parents are separated, children may be handed over to an abusive father for regular contact visits. Thus, the male maintains power and control over the woman he has abused.

A cause for concern

Health and social services in both acute and community settings have established child protection services. However, if as research studies suggest many abused women are overlooked by staff in health services, one must concede that the needs of the children within these families may also be invisible.

Therefore, healthcare practitioners have to be on the alert for female clients in an abusive relationship; ensuring additional protocols are in place to deal with the health and safety of children from these homes.

THE IMMEDIATE IMPACT OF DOMESTIC VIOLENCE ON CHILDREN

Children's responses vary enormously with some children being affected far more than others, and children within the same family can be affected differently. Each child's experience and reactions are unique . . . it will be hard to discern the impacts of living with domestic violence on children, especially as some of the resulting behaviours also occur in children experiencing other forms of abuse and neglect.

(Hester *et al.* 2000: 44)

The list of possible negative effects can appear endless and includes:

- Being secretive, silent and afraid to tell.
- Being protective of their mother and/or siblings, which may lead to them having a maturity beyond their years, whilst other children exhibit regression. Alternatively they may mimic the aggression of the abusive parent and be abusive to the mother and siblings.
- Attitudes to their father or stepfather may be ambivalent, often due to a feeling of confusion.
- Being fearful, hyper-vigilant, mistrustful, anxious and sometimes excessively agitated.
- Experiencing feelings of guilt and helplessness and even thinking that the violence is their fault. This is particularly so if the violent episode follows an argument between the adults that is related to the child.
- Experiencing nightmares, bedwetting, sleep disturbances, eating difficulties leading to weight loss or obesity.
- In some children, long periods of sadness, which may progress to depression.
- In younger children, delay in developmental milestones.
- In contrast in some older children, a very adult way of acting in order to minimize the violence or protect the mother.

In addition Hester *et al.* (2000: 44) found that whilst some children have poor social skills others attain a high level of social skills development with an ability to negotiate difficult situations. A child's ability to acquire sophisticated coping strategies to deal with the on-going abuse should never be underestimated; neither should the child's attachment to the abusive parent which, for some, may continue to be strong.

> **Key point**
>
> It ought to be noted that whilst there is a wide spectrum of possible negative health and social outcomes for children who have lived in an abusive home, not all children manifest adverse characteristics in their later life. We should never underestimate the power of recovery and the resilience of many children, young people or adults, who are able to move forward from the situation.
>
> It is important to remember that some children remain perfectly well adjusted despite living with abuse and that a majority survive within non clinical or 'normal' levels of functioning.
>
> (Mullender and Morley 1994: 4)

POSSIBLE LONG-TERM EFFECTS ON THE CHILD

Nevertheless there are those like Brandon and Lewis who believe that

> The evidence points to the possibility that the cumulative harm from witnessing violence will affect the child's emotional and mental health in future relationships. . . . [U]ntil professionals recognize that when the child sees violence at home there is a likelihood of significant harm, it will not be possible to prevent long-term damage.
>
> (1996: 41)

Child psychologists often hold competing views with regards to the medium- and long-term effects of family violence in later life. This section offers a synopsis of theories in an attempt to facilitate healthcare practitioners in their understanding and future practice.

Kashani and Wesley (1998: 37), summarizing contemporary research, acknowledge that children who have grown up in an abusive home whilst remaining a heterogeneous group, nevertheless have similarities in their responses at the time, and in the future. Children's responses to living in a violent and abusive home can include:

- Pre-school children, particularly boys, seem to be at risk of developing behavioural problems.
- They may express anger and distress in ways viewed by others as inappropriate.
- Carlson (1990) found that adolescent boys from abusive homes were more prone to running away, possibly as a means of avoiding violence against themselves. Similarly, he found adolescent male witnesses to family violence were more apt to use physical violence against their mothers.
- Carlson also found that young males from violent homes had often experienced suicidal thoughts. In a study undertaken by Kashani et al. (1997) they found that juveniles who had committed interfamilial homicide had frequently experienced a significant history of family violence. Moreover, the homicide commonly followed an unsuccessful suicide attempt.

According to the American Medical Association, children of all ages from violent homes:

> may exhibit somatic concerns, including headaches, school avoidance, and abdominal complaints. Pre-school children most often develop stuttering, enuresis, insomnia, and separation anxiety. School age children frequently develop impaired concentration and difficulty staying focused on schoolwork. Older children often manifest aggressive behaviour, with boys being more likely to have such aggressive behavioural problems, while girls are more likely to have somatic concerns. Both sexes often express guilt at not being able to stop domestic violence.
>
> (AMA 1995b: 16)

Studies suggest that routinely the mother does not discuss the violence with her child or children making it harder for them to articulate their thoughts and feelings. Equally, children often avoid talking about their experiences with outsiders for fear of being taken into care, and many retain a degree of loyalty to the abusing father as they have good memories as well as the bad ones.

HEALTHCARE RESPONSE TO CHILDREN IN AN ABUSIVE HOME

The situation for healthcare staff in respect of children can be extremely complex, as there are a number of ways in which the domestic violence may come to their attention. Where the child attends a clinic, or the GP, is visited by the health visitor or is admitted to hospital and there is direct evidence of child abuse, child protection procedures are well established and well documented.

However, where a mother is being abused, but no direct evidence exists that the child is at risk, the healthcare professionals should be cautious in their approach. If the mother fears intervention from other agencies, including the social services, she may be even more reluctant to divulge information of her own abuse. Nevertheless, the child's safety is paramount.

THE SCHOOL NURSE

The Department of Health in 2001 produced a resource pack for school nurses, in which it highlights the need for all school nurses to have adequate knowledge to deal with any children who may come from an abusive home. In particular school nurses are advised to forge links with local domestic violence forums and to work with school staff to ensure they have a working knowledge of the needs of children from a home where their parent is being abused. Specifically school nurses must be aware of, and work within, the child protection guidelines to ensure the safety and well-being of the child. The DoH advises that like other healthcare professionals they should provide information for other staff, and the child's parents, by displaying posters or making literature available.

In addition, the guidelines suggest that a school nurse should:

- lobby for local services that are responsive to family needs; for example, assertiveness and anger management sessions.

- work with other agencies to ensure consistency of approach.
- include domestic violence as part of an SRE (Sex and Relationship Education) plan, ensure ground rules are established and helplines and support services are clearly displayed.
- support local programmes with the police and education welfare in schools and community venues.
- invite the local domestic violence co-ordinator to talk to school staff.
- work with school and primary care to establish clear pathways for when domestic violence is suspected or revealed.

(Department of Health [DoH] 2001: 67)

HEALTH NEEDS OF CHILDREN IN REFUGES

Children in refuges for women victims of domestic violence constitute one of several marginalised groups with poor access to services.

(Webb *et al.* 2001: 210)

On average, 35,000 children annually are cared for in refuges across England and Wales with a similar number being in other temporary accommodation. The fact that many women and children have specific healthcare needs as a result of living in an abusive environment is undisputed; however, their specific health needs whilst they are living in a refuge are rather less well documented. In a recent study undertaken by Webb *et al.* (2001), the healthcare needs of 148 of the 257 children resident in five refuges in Cardiff, over a nine-month period, were studied in detail. The researchers used semi-structured interviews along with a number of validated instruments to assess development milestones, physical, emotional and psychological well-being and general health status.

The study concluded that:

- For safety reasons the mother was unable to have post re-directed to the refuge, therefore appointments for clinics, health visitor visits or GP contact were not forwarded on. Equally going to their usual healthcare centre was not an option, as they did not want anyone to know where they were.
- Whilst each refuge had a named health visitor attached their visits were irregular and often not recorded so that accessing health notes was difficult for the researchers.
- The caseload of each health visitor was already onerous and there did not appear to be additional funding for the supplementary workload within the refuge.
- There are no cost details related to caring for the health of women and children staying in refuges, although it is known that they have specific healthcare needs.
- Of the 68 children tested with the Denver developmental screen six failed the screening and a further seven required a follow-up review, and all 13 children were referred to appropriate services for follow-up.
- The mothers of 113 of the children expressed concern about various aspects of their child's health and after detailed consultation a number were referred on to other healthcare specialists.

- 'Seventy-three referrals were made for 65 children. Thirty-six children were referred to a health visitor; nine to a paediatrician; eight to social services; six to a school nurse; four to a family therapist; three each to child protection, audiology, and enuresis services; and one to a dietician.'

This and other studies concluded that because of the nature of their home circumstances, children are at risk of not receiving regular health screening, and consequently they often do not have their immunizations. Due to the geographical mobility of some of the families, follow-up referrals and appointments may be missed and health needs in the children continue to be unmet.

The time that children spend in refuges provides a window of opportunity to review their health, identify problems, and begin the process of investigation, treatment, and care. The numbers passing through refuges are about half of those in care, on whom a large amount of money is currently being spent in England and Wales.

(Webb *et al.* 2001: 213)

Key point

Primary care trusts (PCTs) have a duty of care to the women and children who seek refuge in temporary accommodation, but their specific needs may remain unmet unless staff are trained to recognize and deal with these. Some PCTs and trusts are sufficiently concerned that they are employing specialist domestic violence healthcare personnel, often senior nurses to deal with the escalating demand.

EFFECTS OF DOMESTIC VIOLENCE ON FUTURE PARENTING SKILLS

Research suggests that the physical and emotional effects of living in an abusive relationship can have a detrimental impact upon the child's future ability to operate as a parent. In contrast, other theorists believe that because of their own experiences some children from abusive homes work extremely hard to ensure they attain positive parenting attitudes and skills. However, what is certain is that children are influenced by their childhood experiences and that to be situated in an abusive and violent home must be exceptionally challenging for any child. There is not the space to address this issue in depth; however, before accepting the notion that abused children do in turn become abusers one needs to ask: How does one explain the many abused children who do not become abusers, conversely what of those that abuse but have never suffered abuse themselves? Such theories do not explain why daughters from an abusive home do not automatically move into abusive adult relationships, or necessarily accept the male domination that perpetuates domestic abuse. 'It is important to remember that children are individuals with unique internal resources which enable them to draw their own conclusions and develop their own interpretations of the world around them' (Corrigan 1998: 15).

FACTORS WHICH MAY MEDIATE THE CHILD'S RESPONSE

Corrigan (1998) argues that children's responses to witnessing their mother being assaulted by their father vary according to the sex, age, and stage of development of the child and their role in the family. Other factors that may influence outcomes are the extent and frequency of the violence, repeated separations and moves, economic and social disadvantage and special needs that a child may have independent of the violence (Jaffe *et al.* 1990). In a recent study that interviewed children from a range of different backgrounds, Mullender (2000) identified that black and Asian children's ability to seek help was significantly influenced by their fears of receiving bad advice and unsympathetic treatment from white organizations.

Studies suggest that the child's stress levels are often associated with the actual and potential threat to their mother and that once she has received support and protection the child may begin to feel safer itself.

CONTINUING PARENTAL CONTACT IN ABUSIVE FAMILIES

The continuing contact between the child and a violent parent remains a contentious issue. Contact orders may be made by a court allowing the father continuing access to the child or children, even when the family has taken residence in a refuge.

Dame Elizabeth Butler-Sloss made a legal judgment on 19 June 2000, in the Civil Appeals court, in ruling on an appeal for a violent man to have continued contact with his children she stated that

> Family judges and justices needed to have a heightened awareness of the long- and short-term effects of domestic violence on children, as witnesses as well as victims, with proper arrangements put in place to safeguard both the child and the residential parent from risk of further physical or emotional harm, as the Report by the Children Act Sub-Committee of the Advisory Board on Family Law, 'Contact between Children and Violent Parents', (December 1999) had made clear.

However, where courts do allow contact visits, to ensure the safety of the child the court may insist that the visit is supervised in a designated area. During the visit, however, it may be possible for a determined father to access sufficient information from the child or children to allow him to subsequently find his missing family. Moreover, evidence indicates a significant number of children may be physically, emotionally and, in extreme cases, sexually abused during unsupervised contact with the father (Hester *et al.* 2000). In addition, there have been cases where the father used the contact visit as an opportunity to disappear with the child or children. Acknowledging that the most dangerous time for the abused woman is after she has left the abusive partner one can see the potential for serious harm in allowing the father to continue to have contact with the child or children.

Humphreys notes that all too often a woman is labelled hostile when fighting for her child not to be subjected to further contact with the abusive father. Other women have been found in contempt of court and even jailed for non-compliance with a contact order. Interestingly, a general acceptance by women to maintain contact between the child and the father in the initial stages of separation has been identified. However, when the matter came to court, 83 per cent of the abused parents did not want contact to be ordered since informal or interim contact arrangements had changed their minds about its viability. The most common reason that is cited by the resident parent for opposing contact is fear for the child's or children's safety and emotional well-being. In these circumstances the social services team, together with other interested persons, can arrange and supervise contact visits. The child, particularly if it is quite young, may have little if any say in whether or not it continues contact with the abusing father. Allowing an abusive man to maintain continuing access to his children is without doubt a major challenge for those professionals involved in the decision-making process.

Key point

It is essential that health professionals equip themselves with the appropriate knowledge and skills crucial to effective and safe assessment of the situation. Confidential records must include a full and accurate account, allowing collaboration and referral to other agencies where necessary.

INTERVENTION STRATEGIES

Children's lives need to be viewed in the round. The complex interplay of risk and protective factors reinforces the need to shift from blaming women for their 'failure to protect' and instead exploring strengths, the potential to create places of safety and support for survivors, and challenges to domestic violence offenders (Women's Aid Federation of England 2001).

According to Women's Aid, any strategies designed to support children in abusive homes should endorse the following principles of good practice:

- Each situation needs to be assessed individually to explore the issues for each child and family.
- Any safety strategies should acknowledge
  - the needs of both the woman and the child or children
  - the effects of the violence in all areas of the child's life or the children's lives
  - the networks which may support the child or children, including those in school and the extended family.

Furthermore, the following questions need to be asked of any interventions:

- Does this practice direct responsibility towards the man and his violence?
- Does the intervention progress the idea that protecting and supporting the child's mother in situations of domestic violence is also good child protection?
- The needs of the woman and the children should be not be conflated – far from it. Separate, but linked, provision is required.

(Women's Aid 2001)

SHARING INFORMATION

Research and experience have shown repeatedly that keeping children safe from harm requires professionals and others to share information: about a child's health and development and exposure to possible harm; about a parent who may need help to, or may not be able to, care for a child adequately and safely; and about those who may pose a risk of harm to a child. Often, it is only when information from a number of sources has been shared and is then put together that it becomes clear that a child is at risk of or is suffering harm.

> The law permits the disclosure of confidential information necessary to safeguard a child or children in the public interest: that is, the public interest in child protection may override the public interest in maintaining confidentiality. Disclosure should be justifiable in each case, according to the particular facts of the case, and legal advice should be sought in cases of doubt.
>
> (Department of Health [DoH] 1999 [S7.32])

GUIDING PRINCIPLES FOR SHARING INFORMATION BETWEEN AGENCIES AND PROFESSIONALS

- Where it is considered necessary to share information with a third person the client should normally be advised.
- Where possible, consent to share information should be obtained from the persons involved.
- However, where circumstances are such that consent cannot be obtained, or it is not in the best interest for it to be known, then sharing information is permissible.
- Agencies should create clear guidelines and protocols related to the confidential sharing of information.
- Where confidential information is shared across agencies without permission, staff should be clear that sharing the information is in the best interest of the child.

The Data Protection Act 1998 states that whilst personal information should be collected fairly and lawfully, it allows for confidential data to be shared without permission of the person involved if for 'the purposes of the prevention or detection of crime, or the apprehension or prosecution of offenders, and where failure to disclose would be likely to prejudice those objectives in a particular case' (Department of Health [DoH] 1999b [S7.34]).

Article 8 of the European Convention on Human Rights is quite clear about the rights of individuals and families to carry out their daily living activities without interference from outside agencies. However, there are certain circumstances when this can be set aside, including when the health and safety of others are thought to be in jeopardy, therefore sharing information related to domestic violence does under certain circumstances fall into this category. For a comprehensive guide on sharing information as it relates to child protection issues, readers are referred to Appendix 4: Data Protection Registrar's checklist for setting up information-sharing arrangements (Department of Health [DoH] 1999a [7.27]).

YOUNG PEOPLE'S ATTITUDES TO VIOLENCE

A recent study undertaken by Mullender highlights an emerging concern about children and young people's attitudes to violence. The study was of 1,300 young persons between the ages eight to sixteen from Bristol, North London and Durham:

- Most knew that domestic violence is common and considered fighting between parents to be wrong.
- The majority felt it was worse for men to hit women as men are stronger.
- Most, especially older children, considered threats to be as bad as actual violence.
- Out of those questioned 75 per cent thought children living with domestic violence could do something practical, i.e. calling the police or telling someone.

Perhaps more importantly, the study showed that:

- Over 75 per cent of 11–12-year-old boys thought that women get hit if they make men angry, and more boys than girls, of all ages, believed that some women deserve to be hit.
- Boys aged 13–14 were even less clear that men should take responsibility for their violence.
- Boys of all ages, particularly teenagers, appeared to have less understanding than girls did, of who is at fault, and more commonly excused the perpetrator.

Healthcare professionals should never lose sight of the fact that whilst there may be no evidence of direct abuse, children and young adults from abusive and violent homes do experience various negative consequences. The seriousness of these may not be manifested for many months or even years, but must never be underestimated. The healthcare professional has a responsibility to respond to the child's actual and potential needs within established frameworks of child protection and confidentiality. For this to succeed, health organizations have to take due care by ensuring that appropriate policies, or protocols, informed by national guidelines, are in place, and that staff are both aware of and able to operate within them.

ASSESSING THE POTENTIAL HARM TO CHILDREN LIVING IN AN ABUSIVE HOME

Corrigan (1998) undertook a literature review of the effects of domestic abuse on children and concluded that the studies highlight three main areas, which appear to be of importance when making an assessment of the impact which domestic violence may have on children. The issues include the individual characteristics of the child; the nature and extent of domestic violence; and the level of support offered to the child (see Fig. 3).

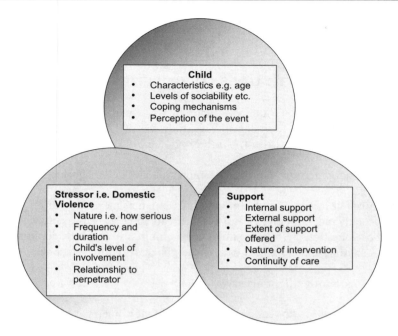

Figure 3 Factors influencing child's response to abuse
Adapted with the permission of NIWAF from S. Corrigan, '"Caught in the Middle". Exploring Children and Young People's Experience of Domestic Violence', Northern Ireland Women's Aid Federation, Belfast 1998

These issues are illustrated in the following:

Child

- characteristics, e.g. age, levels of sociability, etc.
- coping mechanisms
- perception of the event

Stressor in domestic violence

- nature, i.e. how serious
- frequency and duration
- child's level of involvement
- relationship to perpetrator

Support

- internal support
- external support

- extent of support offered
- nature of intervention
- continuity

It is only when we begin to look at these three issues in conjunction that we can understand how a child has suffered, how a child is coping, or the level of support a child needs. It appears that the issue of support is crucial in the overall process of empowering children to come to terms with their own situation. Support may take many forms and be offered by various individuals or agencies working with women and children on a regular basis.

(Corrigan 1998)

Reproduced with permission of Northern Ireland Women's Aid Federation (NIWAF)

DOMESTIC VIOLENCE AND CHILD PROTECTION ISSUES

Domestic violence is likely to have a damaging effect on the health and development of children, and it will often be appropriate for such children to be regarded as children in need. Everyone working with women and children should be alert to the frequent inter-relationship between domestic violence and the abuse and neglect of children (Department of Health [DoH] 1999a).

A major concern in child safety has to be the number of assaults against the woman where the man is not arrested or, if he is, an exclusion order is not made. The children of the family, whilst not necessarily suffering from direct abuse, often become pawns in a potentially dangerous game that leads to emotional distress, if not physical harm. Unfortunately, women are often unlikely to voluntarily seek professional help involving their children for fear that a case conference has negative effects for them. In addition, as the interface between the various agencies, including the criminal and civil justice systems, is complex and often uncoordinated, a child may be placed at serious risk of harm from a violent parent because not all the facts are known at the point significant decisions are made about the child's welfare.

Humphreys (2000) advocates for recommendations of a family case conference to be a part of the evidence at hearings for non-molestation orders and occupation orders. Furthermore, the findings of such case conferences need to be recognized and acted upon when the courts are making decisions in respect of continued parental contact.

RULES OF EVIDENCE

What may or may not be offered as evidence in either a magistrates' court or a criminal court is a complex issue often bound by legal precedence. In response to the government White Paper *Justice for All*, Women's Aid advocates

> that admissible evidence should also include evidence of previous offences, the existence of any civil protection orders or injunctions, AND any concerns about child protection issues, now or in the past. Additional evidence may also be available

from other agencies such as GPs, housing departments, schools, social services or specialist domestic violence services such as Women's Aid.

(Women's Aid 2003: 19)

Specifically, in court proceedings related directly to child abuse, the court should consider receiving evidence from a variety of sources: 'For example, medical evidence and the evidence of professionals such as social services and child psychologists should be admissible in court to support allegations of abuse against children' (Women's Aid 2003: 19). Were these recommendations to be put into place one can see how the records kept by healthcare professionals could become vital evidence in the protection of an abused woman and her child or children.

SOCIAL SERVICES

Under the Children's Act 1989, social workers have a legal duty both to investigate and where necessary to intervene if it appears that a child's welfare is compromised, and having the statutory powers to enact their duty. However, the key to successful intervention is working in partnership with the family, including the children, to resolve the issues, whilst ensuring the child's safety at all times. The social worker is best placed to take the lead in child protection cases, by co-ordinating a multi-agency approach to the issues involved.

Women's Aid (2001) express concern at the fact that some social services departments in the past have sent out a standard letter to families where domestic violence has been identified, advising them that this might be construed as abusive to the children. In effect

> Such a response tends to confirm all the worst stereotypes of the ineffectiveness of social work practice in this area. It fails to differentiate between domestic violence offenders and their victims. Monitoring and surveillance are offered, rather than effective support. This plays into the woman's worst fears, often encouraged by the offender, that the children will be taken into care. The commonly held belief that the woman's needs and safety are not of importance in their own right is confirmed.
> (Humphreys 2000a; Women's Aid 2001)

The Challenge of Partnership in Child Protection outlines 15 basic principles for working in partnership, which are reproduced below.

1   Treat all family members as you would wish to be treated, with dignity and respect.
2   Ensure that family members know that the child's safety and welfare must be given first priority, but that each of them has a right to a courteous, caring and professionally competent service.
3   Take care not to infringe privacy any more than is necessary to safeguard the welfare of the child.
4   Be clear with yourself and with family members about your power to intervene, and the purpose of your professional involvement at each stage.
5   Be aware of the effects on family members of the power you have as a professional, and the impact and implications of what you say and do.

6   Respect the confidentiality of family members and your observations about them, unless they give permission for information to be passed to others or it is essential to do so to protect the child.

7   Listen to the concerns of children and their families, and take care to learn about their understanding, fears and wishes before arriving at your own explanations and plans.

8   Learn about and consider children within their family relationships and communities, including their cultural and religious contexts, and their place within their own families.

9   Consider the strengths and potential of family members, as well as their weaknesses, problems and limitations.

10 Ensure children, families and other carers know their responsibilities and rights, including any right to services, and their right to refuse services, and any consequences of doing so.

11 Use plain, jargon-free language appropriate to the age and culture of each person. Explain unavoidable technical and professional terms.

12 Be open and honest about your concerns and responsibilities, plans and limitations, without being defensive.

13 Allow children and families time to take in and understand concerns and processes. A balance needs to be found between appropriate speed and the needs of people who may need extra time in which to communicate.

14 Take care to distinguish between personal feelings, values, prejudices and beliefs, and professional roles and responsibilities, and ensure that you have good supervision to check that you are doing so.

15 If a mistake or misinterpretation has been made, or you are unable to keep to an agreement, provide an explanation. Always acknowledge any distress experienced by adults and children and do all you can to keep it to a minimum.

(Department of Health [DoH] 1999)
Reproduced with kind permission of HMSO

THE LEGAL FRAMEWORK WITHIN WHICH CHILD PROTECTION OPERATES

A requirement of the *Working Together* document is that police officers attending a domestic violence incident are required to establish where there are children living in the home and ascertain from social services whether these children are on the Child Protection Register. 'It is good practice for the police to notify the social services department when they have responded to an incident of domestic violence and it is known that a child is a member of the household' (Department of Health [DoH] 1999a: 6.38). However, in such circumstances the balance between protecting the child and discouraging the woman from reporting incidents may well lead women to be reluctant to call for help in future, for fear that they may be forced into taking decisions they are not ready to take. In order to ensure that any contact with the woman or family does not exacerbate an already volatile situation, social service staff have to be cautious in their approach. Police attending an incident who have cause to fear for the children's safety at the time of the occurrence are required to contact social services and child protection measures may be instigated immediately. 'Often, supporting a non-violent parent is likely to be the most effective way of promoting the child's welfare. The police and other agencies have defined powers in criminal and civil law that can be used to help those who are subject to domestic violence' (Department of Health [DoH] 1999a: 6.40).

Where action is taken by the police, this can relieve the pressure on the woman, as it then becomes their responsibility to pursue a court case and not the woman's. Thus, there would be little point in the man pressuring her to drop charges as it is no longer her decision.

GUIDE TO GOOD PRACTICE

In responding to situations where domestic violence may be present, consideration should be given to:

- asking direct questions about domestic violence;
- checking whether domestic violence has occurred whenever child abuse is suspected and considering the impact of this at all stages of assessment, enquiries and intervention;
- identifying those who are responsible for domestic violence in order that relevant criminal justice responses may be made;
- providing women with full information about their legal rights and the extent and limits of statutory duties and powers;
- assisting women and children to escape from violence by providing relevant practical and other assistance;
- supporting non-abusing parents in making safe choices for themselves and their children; *and*
- working separately with each parent where domestic violence prevents non-abusing parents from speaking freely and participating without fear of retribution.

Reproduced with permission of HMSO (Department of Health [DoH] 1999a: 6.41)

CHILD PROTECTION ISSUES FOR HEALTH PROFESSIONALS

'All health professionals, in the NHS, private sector, and other agencies, play an essential part in ensuring that children and families receive the care, support and services they need in order to promote children's health and development' (Department of Health [DoH] 1999a: 17). The Department of Health (1999a) requires staff in healthcare settings to play a crucial role in the overall care of children in abusive homes. Healthcare staff and those within other agencies have to be able to recognize when families require support, and contribute where appropriate to family case conferences. There is an expectation that appropriate help is provided by health and social care staff where families have a reduced ability to cope in order to provide adequate and safe childcare. Such intervention may include the provision of support for all vulnerable children and, particularly, those that have been identified as being at specific risk.

Key points

The DoH document makes it quite clear that the government expects all health organizations within the acute and community sectors to:

- provide named professionals, including a senior doctor and senior nurse, within the organization with lead responsibility for setting up and maintaining child protection policies, protocols and procedures.
- ensure all staff working with children have the relevant knowledge and skills related to child protection issues.
- accept that staff working directly with children, are required to undergo a police check to ensure the safety of all vulnerable clients, and specifically children.
- provide adequate training for staff including those outwith the recognized paediatric areas who come into contact with children in need; for instance, staff within Accident and Emergency, midwifery, youth services, etc.
- make a significant contribution to local (and national) multi-professional, multi-agency forums including a domestic violence forum.
- more recently healthcare staff are being asked to recognize the links between domestic abuse and child abuse, to be aware of the relationship between the two and the potential health consequences for children in abusive homes.

Chapter 8

Domestic violence and the legal system

Abused women face a number of problems within the legal process: access to legal representation; lack of specialist services or interpreters for black and ethnic minority women; the trauma of the court process; the lack of training for court staff on the impact of domestic violence on women and children and the reasons why many women stay with or return to a violent partner.

WOMEN'S AID FEDERATION 2002

As one would expect, the impact of the legal system in a range of areas related to domestic violence is both complex and, many would argue, less than perfect for women in abusive circumstances. This chapter explores the law as it relates to the multi-faceted issues including: what can be done to protect the abused; what happens to the perpetrator; and how the legal system can be used to protect the rights of the abused including children within the relationship.

Abused women face several significant challenges within the legal process:

- Access to legal representation: many women are said to feel intimidated by the prospect of seeking legal intervention.
- Costs of legal assistance: not all women are eligible for Legal Aid, so for women who are accountable to their partners for the household budget, seeking legal assistance may appear impossible.
- The trauma of the court process is usually protracted, often adversarial and not renowned for positive treatment of women.
- Lack of specialist services or interpreters for women with disabilities or for black and ethnic minority women increases the trauma of the process.
- Women may find that initiating legal processes exacerbates the violence.
- Legal processes can be protracted which in situations where time is of the essence and could be a source of danger for the woman. It is also difficult for the woman to sustain the secrecy that may be necessary for her to exit the relationship unharmed.

THE EUROPEAN CONVENTION ON HUMAN RIGHTS (ECHR)

According to the Metropolitan Police Service the ECHR under Articles 2, 3 and 8 places police officers under a positive duty to protect both adult and child victims of domestic violence. 'An officer's failure to exercise a power of arrest may leave the victim in immediate danger and the police service open to a legal challenge under the law of negligence within the ECHR' (Metropolitan Police Service 2001: 3). Such a statement leaves one wondering whether, therefore, healthcare professionals need to re-examine their own professional and legal responsibility. Arguably, healthcare organizations and individual staff who fail to provide appropriate care to abused women could equally be said to fail in their duty of care and might therefore be legally held to account.

PROFESSIONAL AND LEGAL RESPONSIBILITY FOR HEALTHCARE PROFESSIONALS

A duty of care to women who are in an abusive relationship

The following section critically reflects upon the potential implications of the Nursing and Midwifery Council's (NMC) *Code of Professional Conduct* (June 2002), for nurses, midwives and health visitors dealing with clients as a result of abuse and/or assault by their partner, past or present.

Section 2.4 affirms that staff must promote the interest of patients and clients including enabling them to gain adequate and appropriate health and social care information. One could therefore argue that the manager of a healthcare venue not displaying the appropriate posters, emergency help-line numbers, or information pertaining to domestic violence is accountable for the deficit. One could also argue that staff who fail to bring the deficit to the manager's attention are equally at fault.

Section 3.2 maintains that one must respect at all times the patients' and clients' autonomy, including their right to refuse treatment. Accordingly, the health professional is required to treat the patients' choices with respect although that choice may lead to continuing violence. Moreover, should the patient or client seek help in the future, but their adverse domestic situation remain unresolved, they retain their right to receive optimal care in a non-judgemental manner.

Section 8 of the code states quite clearly that 'as a registered nurse or midwife, you must act to identify and minimise the risks to patients and clients'. This could call into question the actions of a nurse or midwife who ignores domestic assault as a potential cause or a contributing feature of the client's condition, when to do so might be considered a negligent action. Assessing clients without conceding the risks inherent in abusive relationships may instigate an inadequate risk assessment, thus leading to serious and, on occasion, life-threatening consequences for the client.

The professional bodies for nursing, midwifery and health visiting have all published guidelines relating to the roles and responsibilities for each of the professionals as they relate to clients who have suffered or are suffering as a result of domestic abuse. Thus it can be seen that healthcare staff have a legal, personal and professional responsibility not only to respond to domestic abuse consequences, but to put into place suitable health promotion protocols.

The British Medical Association (BMA)

Through the publication *Domestic Violence: a Healthcare Issue?* (1998) the BMA has made it quite clear to members of the medical profession that they have a duty of care to all patients presenting with illness, or injury related to abuse in an intimate relationship. The BMA believe that medical staff should be involved in the processes of detection, treatment, support, prevention and risk management, in addition to working collaboratively with inter-agency domestic violence forums (British Medical Association [BMA] 1998: 64–6).

The General Medical Council (GMC)

The General Medical Council offers guidance to medical staff on specific aspects related to confidentiality, and to doctors on legal and ethical responsibilities, particularly if the case goes before a court of law. Similarly, various Royal Colleges including that for Obstetricians and Gynaecologists (RCOG) have written specific clinical guidelines for medical staff, which are equally informative for other health professionals.

THE CRIMINAL JUSTICE SYSTEM

What the police can do

Domestic incidents often include behaviour that, providing it is reported to the police, could be dealt with under criminal law. In Mirrlees-Black and Byron (1999), their findings from the British Criminal Survey revealed that when victims in the study were asked to describe the most recent violent incidents:

- Almost two-thirds of domestic assaults involved pushing, shoving and grabbing.
- The assailant kicked, slapped or hit the victim with a fist in nearly half of incidents (47 per cent).
- Throwing objects at the victim was also common (21 per cent).
- Less common were choking, strangling or suffocating, but they did occur in nearly one in ten assaults – most commonly against women.

The study indicated that often women in the study classified as chronically abused had also been forced to have sex, and to have been assaulted with a weapon. Equally, women who are chronically abused often sustain injuries severe enough to warrant medical intervention.

According to the study, victims were injured in 41 per cent of incidents. The most common injuries were:

- bruising (35 per cent of domestic assaults)
- scratches (18 per cent)
- cuts (nine per cent) and broken bones (two per cent).

The study demonstrated that 47 per cent of the women interviewed were injured compared to 31 per cent of the male respondents. Similar studies indicate that abusive women are more prone to using weapons and consequently may cause serious injury to their partner.

Historically there has been a great deal of criticism against police services across the country in their dealings with what were known as 'domestics'. However, many services under the direction of the Home Office have, in the last 10 to 15 years, worked collaboratively with other agencies to provide a service that is much more responsive to and supportive of the needs of the victim.

Domestic violence and criminal law

Domestic violence incidents cross the whole spectrum of criminal offences, in particular as the Metropolitan Police Service (2001: 14) have identified:

- Murder/attempted murder
- Manslaughter
- Rape
- Indecent assault
- Grievous bodily harm/wounding
- Actual bodily harm
- Common assault
- Threats to kill
- Affray
- Threatening behaviour

- Harassment
- Blackmail
- False imprisonment
- Kidnapping
- Criminal damage
- Malicious communications
- Witness intimidation
- Obstructing the course of justice
- Conspiracy to pervert the course of justice

Protection under criminal law

Perpetrators may be prosecuted under the criminal law, and if found guilty be sentenced accordingly. However, reaching the stage of either prosecution or sentencing can be a lengthy and often unsuccessful endeavour. Women's Aid have identified the following as major factors that impact on whether or not abused women co-operate in either an arrest and/or a prosecution:

The difficulties include the following:

- women may be extremely reluctant to give evidence against someone whom they love or have loved, and with whom they share or have shared a home, and who may be the father of their children;
- they may feel under pressure to protect the family reputation;
- black and ethnic minority women may be unwilling to risk community ostracism, and allegations of disloyalty or collusion with police racism;
- women are repeatedly at risk of further violence: waiting times in criminal proceedings are too long and women are frequently left without adequate legal protection whilst waiting for the case to come to court;
- going to court is an ordeal, where women may have to 'run the gauntlet' of their abuser's friends and supporters and hostile defence advocates;
- outcomes at court, when assaults are prosecuted, are not necessarily helpful – usually either a fine (which women often end up having to pay on behalf of their abusive partner) or a suspended sentence, whereupon the man goes home, free to harass again. Imprisonment is rare and often provides only temporary relief as confinement is short.

Moreover, those dealing with victims of domestic abuse should remain aware of the potential dangers:

> Proceeding with prosecution may not however, always be in their best interests. There are a number of practical and emotional difficulties, and prosecution does not guarantee protection or safety in the long term as there may be increased danger of reprisals from a vengeful partner or ex-partner.
>
> (Women's Aid Federation 2000)

Similarly, effective action under criminal law may be undermined by civil proceedings that force women to have continued contact with violent men via the children, and by an uncoordinated approach across the criminal and civil courts.

Many of the violent acts perpetrated by men against women are covered within the existing legal framework for the United Kingdom including that each police officer has the discretion to use his/her powers to intervene, arrest, caution or charge an abusive man (or indeed an abusive woman). An arrest warrant is not required if the police officer has reasonable grounds to believe that the individual is about to commit an arrestable offence, neither is it necessary for an assault to be witnessed by the police officer. Under common law, the Offences Against the Person Act 1861, or the Police and Criminal Evidence Act 1984, one could argue that police officers attending a domestic violence incident have not only the right to arrest but also the responsibility to do so as in any other criminal assault or offence. The police can arrest an individual if they have reason to believe that he or she has committed:

- threats to kill
- criminal damage and public order offences
- assault occasioning actual bodily harm (ABH)
- unlawful wounding or inflicting grievous bodily harm (GBH)
- rape, attempted rape or indecent assault
- attempted murder.

Furthermore, arrests can be made to prevent further injury or to protect 'a vulnerable person or child'. However, whilst the police may recognize the emotional and psychological trauma a woman may be suffering, to cause such conditions is not an arrestable offence. Neither are many minor injuries such as slaps, scratches and injuries that do not leave obvious physical signs of harm. In these cases, the police are often powerless to act in any way other than giving the perpetrator an informal verbal warning. Even when a man is arrested unless the injuries are deemed serious, the police are unable to detain him in custody for a period greater than twenty-four hours, after which he is released on unconditional bail. Whilst attending an incident and determining an appropriate course of action, police need to remain alert to the fact that any action on their part may well exacerbate the violence in the future.

WHAT THE POLICE ARE REQUIRED TO DO

Policing domestic violence in the UK since 1990

In July 1990 the Home Office issued a policy statement known as Circular 60/1990 (with parallel circulars being published in Scotland and Northern Ireland) making strong recommendations as to the way forward for policing as it related to domestic violence.

The main recommendations stated that all police forces (later re-named as police services) were to develop policy statements and strategies based on the belief that domestic violence is a crime as serious as assaults by strangers, and that therefore:

- the primary duty of police is to protect the victim and her children;
- they must take positive action against the assailant;
- they should take positive action in every incident;
- they should recognize that their primary responsibility was rarely to attempt conciliation;
- they should interview the victim separately from the assailant;
- the service should prepare information leaflets for victims;
- an officer should arrange for urgent medical assistance if required;
- the police should escort victims to a place of safety if requested;
- they must consider arresting and charging the assailant and *not* to be affected by the fact that some women withdraw charges;
- they should provide continued support for victims during the pre-trial period;
- local police services should liaise with other agencies, to set up (where practicable) dedicated domestic violence units;
- wherever possible officers should ensure that all offences are properly recorded and not 'no-crimed';
- each police service should make records easily retrievable.

(Home Office 1990)

The roles and responsibilities of domestic violence units are funded and supported by police services, and thus the role of the Home Office is addressed in greater detail in Chapter 9 on multi-agency forums.

THE ROLE OF THE CROWN PROSECUTION SERVICE (CPS)

The role of the CPS is to view all available evidence to determine whether there is sufficient and substantive evidence, which when presented to either a magistrates' court or a jury could result in a conviction. According to the CPS (November 2001), when applied to domestic violence situations they require a prosecution case to meet the following criterion:

Crown prosecutors must first be satisfied that there is enough evidence to provide a 'realistic prospect of a conviction against each defendant on each charge'.

As domestic violence typically occurs in private, and does not always result in personal injury, evidence other than the testimony of the victim may be difficult to obtain. Where the 'victim' is deemed a vulnerable witness, often through fear, the CPS may have difficulty prosecuting. Wherever possible, domestic violence cases are reviewed by a CPS officer with expertise in domestic violence.

Criteria for prosecuting domestic violence incidents

There are a number of factors which taken together influence the CPS's decision to proceed with the prosecution including:

- where there is clear evidence of injury to either the woman or any children in the home;
- where there is a previous history of violence;
- where the police involved in the case believe there is a case to answer and sufficient evidence to proceed;
- any statement made by the woman, even if she subsequently withdraws it;
- any other relevant factors brought to the attention of the CPS.

Some examples of what helps the CPS to decide also include:

- the seriousness of the offence;
- if the defendant used a weapon;
- if the defendant has made any threats since the attack;
- if the defendant planned the attack;
- the effect (including psychological) on any children living in the household;
- the chances of the defendant offending again;
- the continuing threat to the health and safety of the victim or anyone else who is, or may become, involved;
- the current state of the victim's relationship with the defendant;
- the effect on that relationship of continuing with the prosecution against the victim's wishes;
- the history of the relationship, particularly if there has been any other violence in the past;
- the defendant's criminal history, particularly any previous violence.

(Crown Prosecution Service, November 2001)

No witness statement

> In some cases the violence is so serious, or the previous history shows such a real and continuing danger to the victim or the children or other person, that the public interest in going ahead with a prosecution has to outweigh the victim's wishes.
>
> (Crown Prosecution Service, November 2001)

It becomes much more challenging for the CPS if the victim refuses to give a statement or, having done so initially, later withdraws that statement. However, under section 80 of the Criminal Justice Act 1988 the court can compel the victim to give evidence. An alternative to this would be to offer the witness's written testimony to the court without her or his being present (s. 23 of the Police and Criminal Evidence Act 1984). Arguably these two options, whilst not being ideal, offer the witness some protection as she can tell the accused that she gave evidence unwillingly.

> The victim does not have to give evidence to prove that he or she is afraid. This proof can come from someone else, for example, a police officer, doctor, or sometimes it can be seen from the victim's behaviour in court.
>
> (Crown Prosecution Service 1995: 11 [4.18])

Thus, it can be seen that encounters between abused clients and healthcare professionals have to be adequately documented, as the content may prove vital to a future successful prosecution. Complete records of all visits to healthcare settings must be made with a view to possible sharing of information within the boundaries of patient confidentiality. Once a decision to prosecute has been made, the CPS may apply for the accused to be remanded in custody until trial, or to have specific conditions placed on any application for bail. This would occur if the police and/or the CPS had reason to believe that either the victim or others, including the children, remained at risk of further injury, or harassment from the accused. Where bail conditions are imposed, they frequently carry the power to arrest in the event of the conditions being broken, thus enabling the police to act swiftly.

WHAT THE COURTS CAN DO

First, the court can 'bind over'. This is an order that the court can make when it considers that the defendant may offend again in the future. The defendant must agree to behave properly for a specified period. The courts can make a 'binding over order' at the same time as they impose other penalties. However, there must be enough evidence to justify making the order.

Second, the court can make bail conditions including

- banning the defendant from contacting named persons;
- banning the defendant from named places including residences;
- requiring the defendant to pay surety;
- requiring relatives to pay surety;
- requiring the defendant to reside at a specified address;
- requiring the defendant to attend a police station at designated times;
- restricting the defendant in the times he or she is able to be away from home.

Failure to comply with any or all bail conditions may lead to the defendant being held in prison, on remand until the case is heard in court.

HARASSMENT AND STALKING

For countless women the abuse and violence continue long after they have departed the shared home or managed to have their partner removed. In fact, it has long been recognized that the moment at which the relationship is ended is the most vulnerable time for the woman and her children.

- Hester *et al.* (2000: 19) identified that violent males may continue to abuse and harass their female partners using any situation in which they are both going to be present, including at periods of contact with the child.
- Kelly's study (1988) established that 70 per cent of women who left a violent relationship were harassed after separation.
- In Hester and Radford's study (1996) all but 3 of the 53 women interviewed had been assaulted, harassed, or further abused during child contact visits after separation.

Key points

A survey undertaken in 1995 found that nearly 40 per cent of recorded cases involving harassment were where the woman was the ex-partner, or where there had been a close relationship – in other words, post-separation domestic violence (Wallace, 1996).

    In a more recent study it has been estimated that there are 880,000 adults 'stalked' in England and Wales each year: in three out of every ten cases the person doing the stalking is an ex-partner, and in nearly three-quarters of these cases the focus of the persistent and unwanted attention is a woman (Budd and Mattinson 2000).

The study also highlighted that:

- Women (4.0 per cent) more often experienced persistent and unwanted attention compared to men (1.7 per cent).
- Risks were particularly high for young women aged between 16 and 19 (16.8 per cent).
- A further third involved an acquaintance of the victim, including relatives and neighbours (Harris 2000).
- Victims had often endured the unwanted behaviour for a considerable period of time before taking action (Harris 2000).
- Only a third of incidents involved strangers.
- Seven in ten victims stated that they had changed their lifestyle as a result of being harassed.

Whilst the British Crime Survey (1998) estimated that 2.9 per cent of adults had been stalked in the year preceding the survey, this translated in real terms into a total of 900,000 victims in England and Wales, of which an estimated 610,000 were women and the remaining 290,000 were men.

    In law, the act of stalking does not in fact exist. However, it is hoped that the Protection from Harassment Act 1997 may provide more effective protection than has previously been available for abused women, in particular those who no longer live with their abuser. Harassment includes a variety of behaviours including persistence in:

- quietly following the 'victim'
- forcing conversation

- silent, abusive or threatening telephone calls
- silent, abusive or threatening behaviour either to the 'victim' or to the 'victim's' family members or friends
- maintaining a periodic or constant presence in the 'victim's' life, appearing at public venues knowing the person is expected to be there
- physical threats, or acts of physical violence to either the 'victim' or the 'victim's' property
- damaging or destroying property
- sending unwelcome gifts
- ordering unwanted services such as taxis, funeral services, etc.

In 1998, Harris (2000), evaluating the effectiveness of the law in the year following its inception, selected 167 cases that had been presented to the Crown Prosecution Service. The study acknowledged a number of important factors, including:

- The law was used mainly to handle domestic and inter-neighbour disputes.
- In almost all cases, the suspect and victim were known to each other, with 83 per cent of the cases involving intimates.
- By and large, members of the public, including those being harassed by current or past partners, were unaware that legal protection was available.

At first these figures may appear statistically insignificant, until one adds them to the several other factors that contribute to a woman being unable to exit from an abusive relationship.

Key point

It is relatively easy for an individual who has never faced the tangible threat of personal violence to underestimate the degree to which such a fear can control an individual's behaviour.

All healthcare practitioners must recognize and respect that anyone in an abusive relationship past or present may, whilst receiving healthcare, be at risk of continued harassment. The danger is real and must never be dismissed or underestimated by those offering care to the abused individual.

Protection from Harassment Act 1997

The Protection from Harassment Act came into effect in June 1997; its primary aim being to tackle the problem of 'stalking' and harassment, a phenomenon well known to countless women who have left an abusive relationship. The law provides for both criminal and civil legal action to be taken against 'stalking' and harassment, by creating two new criminal offences:

- criminal harassment (s. 2), an offence tried in the magistrates' court;
- an offence involving fear of violence (s. 4), which may be tried by a magistrate or as an indictable offence in the Crown Court.

'An offence is committed if a person, on at least two occasions, is caused to fear that violence will be used against them and the person causing the fear knew this would be the result of his behaviour' (Home Office circular 34/1997, in relation to the Protection from Harassment Act 1997). Conduct in this instance includes abusive and threatening verbal behaviour as well as physical intimidation. Harassment under s. 2 is an arrestable offence, whilst being found guilty of causing another to fear violence under s. 4, may lead to up to five years' imprisonment. If an offender is convicted of either of these offences, there is an additional measure for protection: a restraining order can also be granted by the court, prohibiting the offender from further similar conduct. A breach of such an order is again a criminal offence, which may lead to imprisonment.

An extension of the 1997 Act under s. 3, allows for additional civil law action enabling the victim to claim for any financial losses, and for any stress and distress caused by the harassment. Under the civil law there is also a new injunction for prevention of harassment for those who are not eligible under the Family Law Act 1996. According to the Women's Aid web site (2002):

> In particular, criminal proceedings resulting in a conviction mean that a restraining order can be attached. Restraining orders can provide the same protection as injunctions under the civil law but may be more effective as they carry stronger penalties . . . action under the criminal law, coupled with restraining orders, may avoid the problem of the costs of legal aid for civil remedies, in those cases where women do not need to apply for injunctions to exclude their abuser from the property.

The success or failure of legislation is typically determined by the number of abused persons reporting incidents and the various response approaches adopted by local police services. In 2000, the Home Office published a series of guidelines, 'Reducing Domestic Violence . . . What Works?', aimed at improving practice across diverse departments and agencies including the police, health and social services, local council services, and voluntary organizations. Perhaps not surprisingly it was found that successful implementation is spasmodic and varies across regional boundaries. Furthermore, a study of the 1998 BCS figures indicates that whilst victim and witness intimidation in Britain is not widespread 38 per cent of those women who had been intimidated (152 in total) were related to domestic violence cases (Tarling et al. 2000).

PROTECTION UNDER CIVIL LAW

> Abused women face a number of problems within the legal process: access to legal representation; lack of specialist services or interpreters for black and ethnic minority women; the trauma of the court process; the lack of training for court staff on the impact of domestic violence on women and children and the reasons why many women stay with or return to a violent partner.
>
> (Women's Aid web site 2002)

In addition to protection from the criminal courts, women can, finances allowing, have recourse to legal solutions in the civil courts. However, the process can be lengthy, expensive and often unsuccessful. Professional advice should be sought from a local solicitor, the Citizens Advice Bureau or the Women's Aid local refuge. Other organizations such as the Domestic Violence Intervention Programme (DviP), iVillage, or the Metropolitan Police Service (MPS), to name but a few, offer comprehensive advice either via their web site or in publications available from their respective head offices. A list of useful organization names, addresses, contact numbers and, where available, web pages, is available in Appendix 1.

> Over the last 20 years, the need for a better protection from domestic violence under the civil law has been highlighted through a number of reports and enquiries; research has shown that injunctions and protection orders were more often breached than not, and that enforcement was virtually impossible.
>
> (Women's Aid Federation web site 2000)

One of the challenges for women wishing to seek legal assistance through the civil authorities can be the potential cost. Since the changes to eligibility for Legal Aid in 1997, there is evidence to suggest that women find themselves excluded from such financial help.

In addition, according to the Women's Aid Federation web site (2000):

> following the introduction of revised criteria in 1997 for applications for injunctive protection: these include the requirement that a warning letter should have already been sent to the home [of the perpetrator], a measure that women might refuse for safety reasons. The new criteria also appear to be partly connected to an assumption that civil protection is only required if criminal law measures are not in place.

PART IV OF THE FAMILY LAW ACT 1996

> Part IV [of the Family Law Act 1996] deals with rights to occupy the matrimonial home, occupation orders and non-molestation orders. It also includes amendments to the Children Act 1989 concerning interim care orders and emergency protection orders. The provisions offer a single consistent set of remedies which will be available in all courts with family jurisdiction.
>
> (Department of Health, September 1997)

This section offers the reader an overview of the main elements of this Act. For those directly involved in, for instance, child protection, further reading is needed. Amongst the available literature for staff and clients, healthcare organizations should include a list of expert personnel and local agencies where essential information pertaining to the client's legal rights can be obtained. Multi-agency forums often include within their membership a local firm of solicitors to act as advisers to the group.

What the Act seeks to do is:

- It has provided a single consistent set of remedies available to all courts which have family jurisdiction.

- It has extended the range and powers of 'Occupation orders' and 'Non-molestation orders'.
- It has introduced a wider range of potential applicants (previously some legislation was confined to heterosexual married couples).
- In cases of proved violence, powers of arrest are more readily available.
- The Act seeks to extend the previous definitions and understanding of concepts related to domestic violence. In so doing it has recognized that, for instance, molestation goes beyond the physical act.

(F. Smith 1998)

The Act seeks to include individuals who have hitherto had little if any legal redress in domestic violence situations, including couples who cohabit, lesbian and gay couples, and non-cohabiting couples.

Other changes that have been implemented include:

- Most orders now carry with them the powers of arrest.
- Occupation orders may be granted in the absence of the perpetrator from the court (*ex parte*).
- Occupation orders have greater flexibility as they range from short- through medium- to longer-term.

Occupation orders [s. 62(2)]

Sections 33 to 41 of the Family Law Act 1996 set out provision for occupation orders. Such orders decide who is allowed to occupy the home and who in certain circumstances can direct another party to leave the home. The terms of the order and the factors to be considered vary according to whether or not the applicant is entitled to occupy the property and their relationship to the other party or parties. Under certain circumstances, children may now apply, with leave of the courts, for similar orders from the High Court. Determining the rights of the various parties can involve complex legal argument and is therefore outwith the domain of most healthcare practitioners. Nevertheless, when dealing with clients in domestic violence situations a practitioner may need to be cognizant of the potential legal rights of the client and their family. It is particularly relevant for those practitioners working in child protection, or working with the homeless and immigrant women.

One of the most significant changes that has occurred as a result of the Family Law Act, is that it has effectively expanded the range of persons who may seek legal redress in domestic incidents. Such individuals are referred to as 'Associated Persons' [s. 62(3)].

Non-molestation orders [s. 42(1)]

Section 42 sets out provisions for non-molestation orders. Such orders are defined as containing either or both of the following:

- provisions prohibiting the respondent from molesting another person who is associated with the respondent (e.g. a spouse or former spouse or a cohabitant).
- provisions prohibiting the respondent from molesting a relevant child.

The court may make an order under this section in any family proceedings if it considers it to be of benefit (including to any relevant child) and may do so of its own motion. This provision also may be used in proceedings where an emergency protection order has been made under s. 44 of the Children Act, which includes an exclusion requirement (Department of Health [DoH] 1997b). The orders have been extended to include lesbian or gay people who are living, or have lived, in the same household.

In the 1990s, major steps were made by a variety of policy-making organizations, agencies and professional bodies to improve the service to those who live in fear of violence from someone with whom they once shared, or still share, an intimate relationship. However, a great deal of work remains to be done in this field to ensure there is greater co-operation amongst the numerous organizations and agencies which collectively provide services.

Chapter 9

Multi-agency approach to domestic violence

> Partnership working is essential to providing a comprehensive response to the wide range of needs that domestic violence survivors may have.
>
> (Home Office 1999)

The word 'multi-agency' is used throughout this chapter, which discusses the perceived strengths and weaknesses of a multi-agency, inter-agency approach; inter-agency, multi-professional and inter-professional groups are inclusive within this usage.

Whilst it is generally agreed that greater co-operation and co-ordination between agencies provide more effective and responsive services across a range of health and social care initiatives, significant challenges exist for those involved. Not least are the inequitable power dimensions between the collaborating individuals and agencies and the manner in which this differential can impact upon the decision-making processes. For more than a few professional and voluntary bodies to agree guiding principles or mutual philosophies to meet individual and collective needs, requires a considerable degree of negotiation and mutual understanding. For example, each agency, individual or organization has its own values and beliefs that define its specific agenda and consequently there are times when these militate against a harmonious, collaborative process.

This chapter explores the roles and responsibilities of a range of agencies and organizations that collectively seek to make a difference to the women and children they endeavour to serve. Additionally, the role of the major policy-making institutions and organizations is explored.

THE PURPOSE OF INTER-AGENCY DOMESTIC VIOLENCE FORUMS

The needs of a woman in a violent and abusive relationship and those of her family tend to be very complex and inter-related. Seeking healthcare intervention for physical injuries or the mental health abuse consequences is in itself limited if the woman has to return to the perpetrator. For interventions to be successful, individuals, organizations and groups with a shared interest have to operate co-operatively to be effective. In doing so they can:

- identify common goals that seek to acknowledge women's needs and preferences, which are achieved more effectively through collaboration;
- develop good practice that works towards the provision of co-ordinated services, which complement and enhance that which can be achieved by individual organizations;
- facilitate the development and operation of sound, safe policies across agencies;
- offer services that have the needs of the women at the centre of policy-making;
- provide expert knowledge to one another and to others outwith the forum;
- to work with other multi-agency forums to extend good practice across the country;
- to act collectively to inform, improve and evaluate national policy decision-making.

MULTI-AGENCY FORUMS: BEST PRACTICE?

Over the years, various studies have been undertaken to identify factors that should exist if multi-agency work is to have significance, and the following features appear often within the literature. Most importantly, the woman's voice must be heard, as all too often the service user, the abused woman, either has no voice or one that is so small it is all but ignored by those who think they 'know best'. Moreover, to succeed, members of a multi-agency forum must strive to maintain consistent representation and clear lines of account-ability; failure to do so leads to an inconsistency in the service offered. Consequently, individual members become disenfranchised from the services being offered; but more importantly, inconsistency impacts on what can be offered to the clients.

Principles of good practice for multi-agency forums

In addition to the above, any multi-agency, domestic violence forum should seek to:

- combine input from a variety of practitioners with commitment from senior managers and policy-makers
- ensure a central role for Women's Aid and the refuge movement
- value and support the contributions of voluntary organizations, including local specialist women's organizations, as equal partners
- support participation by women survivors and their children
- be seen as part of participating members' core work, not an 'add-on' extra
- have resources to support a full-time paid co-ordinator
- move beyond networking to develop guiding principles, shared objectives and practical action plans
- resist the temptation to take on too much at once
- recognize and respond to issues of diversity
- balance innovation with support for established programmes
- ensure real improvements in service provision arising form their joint efforts.

(Adapted from Young *et al.* 2001)

Hague (2000) observes how a multi-agency approach to tackling domestic abuse forms the cornerstone of the present government's strategy to deal with what has been designated by the Department of Health, a major public health issue. Hague further notes that one weakness of current systems is an acute shortage of financial support to existing schemes, limiting the groups' potential to explore new initiatives or adequately evaluate those currently in existence. Frequently, work done in these areas depends on the goodwill of those who place it high on their personal and, on occasion, professional, agenda.

> While many agencies are enthusiastic about the potential of inter-agency work, increased co-ordination is of little use if the resources and services are not in place.
>
> (Hague 2000: 275)

Hague further notes how multi-agency initiatives generally are perceived by many to be the preferred option for professionals to deal with a variety of social problems and issues. For example, health and social work colleagues are finding their individual professional boundaries merging in areas that include child protection, care of clients with mental health needs, and care of individuals with learning difficulties and adults with disabilities, significant areas of practice that have been enhanced by a bi-partite approach. Increasingly with the emphasis of healthcare refocusing away from the acute services to a community service provision, the need for collaborative working practices increases exponentially. Unfortunately, more than a few multi-agency initiatives, in a range of practice areas, have either failed to meet their primary objectives or, having met them, fail to maintain the momentum over time.

In the national 'Break the Chain' programme, the Home Office (2000b) published a comprehensive guide advising multi-agency staff on the components that constitute good practice. The guide provides direction for all statutory organizations and forms the basis for subsequent government directives and projects related to domestic abuse, it is recommended reading for those readers requiring more detail on work in the field of individual agencies.

WHO IS INVOLVED?

Both statutory and voluntary sector agencies, including Women's Aid and the refuge movement, ought to be involved in any multi-agency, multi-professional forum. The majority of experts within the field advocate multi-agency co-operation at local level believing that use of the services is optimized when policies and practices are in harmony.

> Virtually all local authorities had a domestic violence forum covering their area. However, evidence from the case studies suggested that the key local authority departments did not always attend regularly, or sent relatively junior members of staff, which affected the extent to which fora could influence policy.
>
> (Home Office 2000a)

In writing for the Home Office 2000a, Hague identifies that women's refuges and the police are most frequently members of any local forum. However, whilst many forums were established by the police she points out that it is not necessarily good practice for the police to continue to lead the groups once established. Hague notes that the relationship between the police and other members, especially those related to the specific needs of women from minority groups, has not always been harmonious. Therefore, for the police to take the lead role in the running of the group may lead to uncomfortable power differentials that inhibit an effective working relationship between its members. It is essential that those representatives on the group have sufficient power, or access to those within their organization with the power to formulate and operationalize any policy decisions made by the group.

PURPOSE OF THE MULTI-AGENCY FORUMS

Many of the established groups emerged and developed in an ad hoc manner. Some groups initially formed to network and support each other in local initiatives running with little external financial support. However, most have evolved into more formalized groups whose main objectives are related to the improving of the service to, and safety of, women and children who are in abusive relationships. Whilst there are no definitive standards and protocols for setting up and operating a multi-agency group, it is generally recognized that the following principles should be adhered to.

Key points

The group should have as wide a representation as possible, but should not be so large that individual members feel intimidated by the power differentials. Each member of the forum holds their own personal beliefs and values, whilst others also represent those of their organization. Therefore, the members may on occasion need to agree to differ on individual points whilst recognizing that they are attempting to seek shared solutions, or formulate guiding principles for implementation at an organizational level. Consequently, compromise is a regular 'visitor' to the decision-making process. An individual group member requires an understanding and an acceptance of the work of other members and the organizations they work for. In addition, the group should respect the differences of others.

For any group to be effective, it requires:

- sufficient funding to establish and maintain the work of the group, including access to additional funding for new initiatives, research and process evaluation;
- that the person who is to chair the group be established and decisions agreed as to the period it is to be for, and the process for choosing a new chair. Authors such as Hague (2000) have suggested that it is inappropriate for the police to chair such a forum.
- an agreed working definition of domestic violence and domestic abuse;
- that terms of reference be negotiated and agreed by the group membership;
- clear and, where possible, unambiguous aims and objectives;
- that specific objectives supported by action plans 'are regularly reviewed, updated and usually time-limited so that participants can organize their workloads' (Hague 2000);

continued

- that each member equires adequate time to support the team both at meetings, and by taking the work back into their organization;
- that local policies should where possible mirror those of a wider, even national agenda whilst reflecting the specific needs of the local client group;
- that established groups across the country need to work more towards exploring and researching initiatives that have potential to be used over a wider provision than locally. Similarly, evaluative studies might be enhanced if the focus of the studies had some shared elements including a definition of domestic violence.

THE IMPORTANCE OF SERVICE USERS IN MULTI-AGENCY WORK

The significant role of service users in all aspects of domestic violence intervention is well documented. Unfortunately, the research consensus indicates that whilst there are pockets of excellent practice across the country, repeatedly reality does not meet expectations. Providing a service to meet the needs of the user groups would appear to be the most appropriate way to progress; unfortunately, as sometimes happens with 'helping' agencies, the 'providers' set an agenda based on the premise that they know best. Hague *et al.* (2001: 2), in their study into multi-agency initiatives, discovered that: 'A wide-scale commitment in principle to service user participation emerged, though few inter-agency forums, or domestic violence projects associated with the statutory sector, had concrete consultation mechanisms in place.' In their study, perhaps not surprisingly, the women identified far greater participation in decision-making processes within refuges and women's groups than they did within domestic violence forums. Despite crucial changes in services for abused women over the last decade, still many of the women interviewed felt marginalized, and powerless within the decision-making at policy level. The women reported that when they approached an agency either they were disbelieved, or they found their complaint was minimized. Some women reported intervention strategies that left them feeling extremely unsafe. Within the study, the service found to have improved the most was the police service, especially where dedicated domestic violence officers were appointed. The research respondents considered there had also been noticeable improvements within housing agencies whilst:

> Overall, poor health service ratings (25 per cent) gave cause for concern, while the courts and the Benefits Agency (at 13 per cent and 12 per cent respectively) emerged as the organizations least likely to respond appropriately or to understand the reality of domestic violence.
>
> (Hague *et al.* 2001: 3)

Without exception, the service viewed in the most positive light was the refuge services and associated women's support groups although the respondents emphasized the constant under-financing of these establishments. The study concluded that without the voices of the women who use the services, multi-agency provision continues to be inadequate and in some instances inappropriate and potentially unsafe.

THE WOMEN'S AID MOVEMENT

The first Women's Aid Federation, established in 1974, was built on the work of individuals across the country working to provide support and shelter for women in abusive relationships. Within a three-year period, forty refuge groups had become one hundred.

Harwin *et al.* (1999: ch. 3), identifies the constant struggle that existed between the work of the federation and others in the field such as social workers, police and members of the criminal justice system. 'There were of course some positive responses from the very beginning, but these were ad-hoc and largely dependent on the interest, concern, or commitment of isolated individuals working within these agencies' (Harwin 1999: 29). Harwin illustrates how in the early years there was little common ground between the feminist activists of the early refuge movement and the rigid, strictly hierarchical male-dominated key organizations and policy-makers of that time. However, the relationship between Women's Aid and other statutory organizations began changing in the late 1980s as they played an essential role in establishing local multi-agency forums. Over time, the Women's Aid movement had grown in both strength and stature, as its members became leaders in the field in establishing working programmes that crossed organizational boundaries. Women's Aid, and other women's groups, currently act in a major advisory capacity on national strategic policy-planning programmes related to domestic violence. In addition, they play an important role in the international arena by awareness-raising and campaigning for women's rights and safety. Nevertheless, the strength of the role of individual local branches of Women's Aid in multi-agency forums can still on occasion be problematic. Often the power differential within local groups is such that the larger organizations set and run the agenda.

Harwin *et al.* (1999: 35) maintains that despite the significant improvement in the working of multi-agency forums, there are still groups that suffer from lack of financial support, lack of co-ordination and inadequate commitment from the local authorities. This is compounded when, within the individual organizations, the workforce may lack appropriate and on-going training in domestic violence issues, so that policy does not become practice.

For healthcare practitioners, a link between the health organization and the local refuge is essential if the women identified within a healthcare setting are to be offered appropriate and on-going care. Studies have identified that in many instances where multi-agency forums are established, healthcare representation can be noticeable by its absence. Arguably, it is unsound practice for any organization to establish an in-house group to write policies and protocols related to the identification, assessment, management and evaluation of domestic violence without consulting with their local refuge, and local women's group. A central role of the Women's Aid Federation, is to advise and support any local (or national) healthcare initiatives especially those related to awareness-raising and training.

Women's and community organizations

Kelly and Humphreys (2001) emphasize the need to recognize that outreach and advocacy programmes within the community are essential rather than marginal responses to domestic violence.

> Outreach services broadly comprise responses that support domestic survivors in their homes and communities providing accessible points where information about service provision, and follow up contact are available. Advocacy incorporates a similarly wide range of activities.
>
> (Kelly and Humphreys 2001: 239)

Initially, many of the support services were established within the refuge system; however, in recent years there has been a proliferation of 'helping agencies' including women's advocate groups. Humphreys and Kelly found the identifying of outreach services was not without its problems, noticeably within government documents related to domestic violence where the terminology is used but few specific resources appear to be ring-fenced for such activities. What is not in dispute is the identified need for a range of community services that are user-focused, easy to access and adequately supported and funded by local and national funding bodies. All too often outreach services, including those for abused women, are closed when monies are short, leaving the most vulnerable members of society at increasing risk of harm.

Outreach programmes often emerge when the needs of specific groups are not adequately met by the more mainstream agencies. A study in 1998 demonstrated that the needs of ethnic minority women could best be met through local advocacy and outreach programmes. The same applies in other locations to women with disabilities, women with mental health needs, women in rural areas and women who are governed by the one-year immigration rule (Kelly and Humphreys 2001). More recently, with the influx of women seeking asylum from their country of origin there is a recognized need in some localities for outreach programmes to support these women; many of whom suffered multiple rapes and continued violence from the occupying forces.

Women's Aid refuges and specialist refuges

There exists a national network of women's refuges across the United Kingdom, which work co-operatively to support all women in violent situations. Any local multi-agency group should seek to meet the needs of women from specific religious and ethnic minority groups. For example, in the London borough of Greenwich, there are specialist groups for Asian women, African and Afro-Caribbean women, as well as for women with disabilities, all of which can represent the specific needs of the women they work for.

The next section demonstrates the serious effects of domestic violence and abuse on the lives of many women who are forced to leave their homes. The statistics shown are designed to highlight the extent and seriousness of the problem.

The number of refuges and the funding for them has changed over time. In 1998, when Levison and Kenny undertook to research homelessness as a direct result of domestic violence they identified that, at that time, there were a total of 409 refuge properties in England alone and that:

- 129 (32 per cent) were owned by local authorities;
- 234 (57 per cent) were owned by registered social landlords (RSLs);
- 21 (five per cent) were owned by refuge groups;
- 10 (two per cent) were privately owned;
- 7 (two per cent) had other types of owner; and for
- 8 refuges (two per cent), the owner was not reported.

Furthermore, the study showed the numbers of women and children using the refuges and the lengths of stay.

Key points

The number of women in refuges

'There were 2,256 women resident in refuges (in England) at the end of February 2000, almost three-quarters (72 per cent) had children with them or were pregnant. Almost half (46 per cent) of children resident at this time were under five years, 38 per cent were aged between five and ten years and 16 per cent were over ten' (Levison and Kenny 2002: 15).

A total of 19,910 women and 28,524 children were accommodated in England during 1997–8, with at least a third of the women leaving the refuge within a week and a significant number within a month.

At least 20 per cent of the women, who sought refuge, were thought to have returned home during this period.

DOMESTIC VIOLENCE AND HOMELESSNESS

Recent statistics illustrate how the major cause of homelessness for women, between the ages of 30 to 49, was domestic abuse (BBC on-line 1999). A report by the charity Crisis established that 63 per cent of homeless women in this age group became homeless because they were being abused at home, and that they had been forced to leave. The report confirms that over half the women had slept rough, the majority on more than one occasion – despite the fact that this made them vulnerable to rape and abuse. Several of the women interviewed revealed how they had resorted to drugs and alcohol to blot out the dangers. The report, 'Out of Sight, Out of Mind?', interviewed 77 homeless women across the UK in an effort to learn why, when homelessness is in general decreasing, the number of women in hostels or on the streets is increasing. Countless women in the study found the hostels threatening and thus they preferred to sleep on the streets. More than a few of the women interviewed had multiple health problems including those associated with drugs, alcohol misuse and mental illness.

Mullender (1996: 57) reveals housing to be one of the foremost reasons why women stayed in violent and abusive relationships, knowing that they had little chance of getting alternative accommodation if they left. Mullender confirms that a woman who becomes homeless because of needing to escape a violent partner faces a multiplicity of challenges. These may include unhelpful and, on occasions, hostile staff in housing and benefit offices, to the point where women have little alternative but to return home. In recent years, although women's legal rights to housing have been strengthened through legislation, nevertheless many women are left with no alternative other than to return to an abusive home. The plight of a woman in fear for her life, who needs to seek accommodation in another borough, or another part of the country, is even more fraught with difficulties.

According to Women's Aid (2001):

> The local authority has a temporary, but renewable, two year duty to house certain applicants, people who fit all the following criteria: homeless or threatened with homelessness; eligible for assistance; in priority need; not intentionally homeless; unable to access other 'suitable accommodation'; and who have a local connection with the area.

In spite of this, women do not have the automatic right to permanent re-housing which they have to re-apply for within a two-year period. As with any legislation the process is often complex and confusing, therefore healthcare practitioners ought to be in a position to offer clients an emergency help-line number for expert advice related to homelessness. If the woman is unable to return home for fear of further violence then, with her permission, the healthcare professional can facilitate access to the nearest women's refuge, and/or police.

Local authorities are required on occasion to re-house women who have been made homeless due to violence and abuse within the home. Moreover whilst determining the woman's right to housing or re-housing *Living without Fear* (Home Office 1999) states that the local housing authority policies are required to take the following directives into account:

- Psychological abuse may be an acceptable reason for an individual being forced to leave their home and therefore they may have the right to be re-housed.
- 'The law requires that applicants who are homeless because of domestic violence and who apply to an authority in an area where they do not have a local connection must not be referred back to the authority in their home area (or any other area) if they would be at risk of domestic violence there' (s. 2c.iii.2).
- Women who have been made homeless and either do not have children and/or are not pregnant may have the priority right to be re-housed.
- Women fleeing domestic violence who decline to return to their home under the protection of a non-molestation order or other court order should not be considered to be either not homeless or intentionally homeless on the basis that it is safe for them to return.
- Local housing authorities must give positive consideration to women who have had to move away from other authorities to escape the violence.
- Sympathetic treatment is given to victims of domestic violence, for example, where there are rent arrears or a need to fit new locks.
- Eviction action should be taken against local authority tenants whose partner has fled the home because of domestic violence perpetrated by the tenant.

(Home Office 1999: 11)

Housing associations and housing agencies work in collaboration with the local authority to meet local housing needs including those who have been made homeless due to domestic violence. Healthcare professionals ought to be capable of offering the client local contact numbers and where possible information sheets.

In the government report on housing provision for households experiencing domestic violence in England produced by Levison and Kenny and published by the Deputy Prime Minister's office (2002) key findings were that in some areas, there are 'examples of good partnership working and the effective integration of accommodation and other services provided by local women's refuge groups into local service provision' (2002: 10). However, in major areas the report found that 'there is still a lack of women-only provision and a lack of recognition of the range of both accommodation and support needs that women and their children experiencing domestic violence have'.

The Homelessness Act 2002 required all housing authorities to adopt a homelessness strategy by July 2003 and keep it under constant review. Therefore, it is anticipated that the provision for individuals and families made homeless as a result of domestic violence should significantly improve within the next few years.

> [W]here applicants are experiencing domestic violence but do not automatically have priority need because of dependent children or pregnancy, the housing authority must assess whether they are vulnerable and have a priority need as a result of the violence.
>
> (Levison and Kenny 2002: 13)

The study was undertaken primarily to establish the degree and type of housing accommodation available to individuals and families made homeless as a consequence of domestic abuse. The main findings included the following. At the time of the study, nine out of the ten local authorities were using temporary accommodation for people made homeless as a direct result of domestic violence. In March 1999 there were an estimated 7,177 households who had been accepted as homeless because of domestic violence and who were living in temporary accommodation, including approximately 1,067 in refuges. Of these:

- 31 per cent of those housed on a temporary basis were living in local authority or housing association accommodation;
- 25 per cent were staying temporarily with friends or relatives;
- 15 per cent of homeless households were residing in refuges;
- 13 per cent were in hostels;
- six per cent were in bed and breakfast accommodation;
- not all the women in the refuges had registered as homeless for a variety of reasons: they make up the other ten per cent.

Perhaps not surprisingly, the report noted the lack of special facilities nationally for women with mental health difficulties, and with learning disabilities and other disabilities. Refuges to meet the needs of particular ethnic groups were, as one might expect, situated in specific geographical local authorities, mainly in areas with high ethnic populations from specific groups. Research often shows that women from various ethnic groups may have serious challenges when seeking alternative housing, especially those with non-confirmed immigration status.

Any housing strategy should, where possible, consider the wishes of the family, their safety, which must be paramount, and the availability of alternatives. If children are involved, it is crucial for the parent to accept that the children's safety is the priority and decisions are made accordingly. However, the 'professional' would be ill advised to disregard a woman's assessment of the anticipated scale of her partner's violence and his ability to seek out information of their whereabouts.

The role of the domestic violence forum is to ensure its members work in partnership to determine the nature of the housing problem locally, and then, by listening to the women's voices, to co-operate with each other to design a supportive and comprehensive intervention strategy. In addition, the forum can adopt an active role to ensure that local and national government are advised of the nature of the problem, and of the progress of local initiatives through reports and research.

THE POLICE

Most police services throughout the UK now have named officers in place, or domestic violence units (DVUs) to deal with all and any such cases. The police often play an important co-ordinating role in any forum, as they work directly with and through each agency and organization. 'The police are the only 24-hour emergency protection service available in every locality to respond to violent attacks. Therefore, they are uniquely situated to provide immediate aid to victims of domestic violence' (Morley and Mullender 1994: 18). A review of police activities related to domestic assaults in the UK, during the 1970s through to the 1980s, reflects the belief at that time that such incidents were a private matter, and therefore not ordinarily within the police domain. As a rule, police only intervened when serious injury had occurred, or it was apparent that the conflict would recur once the police had left the scene. According to Morley and Mullender (1994), reviewing the literature on police activity in domestic violence revealed that previous studies inferred arrest served a number of positive functions. For example, some studies concluded that arrest provided immediate protection for the abused by removing the assailant in addition to which, it sent a message to the assailant, victim and community that domestic violence is a serious crime. Moreover, arrest gave the police a tangible product for work that is conventionally viewed as a waste of time, giving it greater credibility. More fundamentally, however, arrest is believed to deter offenders from repeating their violence, that is, to have a direct preventive effect.

However, when this trial was reproduced in other locations arrest did not prove to be a consistent deterrent. Morley and Mullender (1994) summarizing established that in fact arrest in itself might not be the deterrent it was hoped. The whole criminal justice system needs to respond effectively to violent crime, moreover in some instances there exists the danger that following arrest the angry male partner may seek serious retribution on his female partner. Morley and Mullender concluded that:

> Jurisdictions where policies appear to have produced positive effects on practice are ones where the CJS is an integral part of a comprehensive, co-ordinated community

response, and *accountable* to women through continued internal and independent monitoring.

(1994: 21)

Thus it signified a need for a co-ordinated and effective criminal justice system to protect women and children from violence within the home.

Other police initiatives, including the MPS 'Enough is Enough' campaign published in December 2001, demonstrate that co-ordinated and prolonged campaigns across agencies can make effective changes. However, the impetus can be hard to maintain over time and once begun projects often require systematic reviews and modifications.

Grace (1999: 211) offers a synopsis of a study undertaken between 1992 and 1994 on the relationship between the police at that time and other agencies. She concluded that in some locations the overall attitude of the police had not improved significantly despite the fact that the role of the DVUs had expanded and some individual officers had made progress.

Domestic violence units (DVUs)

Since their inception in 1987, DVUs in some areas have had noticeable positive effects whilst others have provided a mediocre service.

> A particularly notable advance has been the creation of domestic violence units [DVUs]. The first was established in Tottenham, London in 1987. By the end of 1992, DVUs existed in 62 out of the 69 Divisions in the Metropolitan Police, and in 20 of the 42 other police forces in England and Wales. (Home Affairs Committee 1993a: para 23).
>
> (Morley and Mullender 1994: 19)

Whilst in some police areas a DVU has an important role to play, and is reasonably well staffed and supported by senior management, in other areas the 'unit' may be one officer and a telephone answermachine. A recent criticism of the work of the DVUs or the DVOs is that they may receive little support from their colleagues within the service:

> However, a recent study (Plotnikoff and Woolfson, 1998) showed that communication between DVOs and other police officers was not always good. It found that DVOs could feel marginalised and some believed that domestic violence was regarded as having a low priority within their forces.
>
> (Home Office 1999: 2b.iii.3)

The roles and responsibilities and a critique of the criminal and civil justice system, including the Crown Prosecution Service (CPS), has been covered in more detail in Chapter 8.

The police and child protection issues

When called to a domestic violence incident the police have a responsibility to ascertain whether there are children in the home, and establish any immediate risk to their safety.

In the *Working Together to Safeguard Children* document (Department of Health [DoH] 1999: s. 6.39), police are required to adopt systems whereby they can check with the local social services to determine whether any children in the home are on the Child Protection Register. The police are advised to notify social services of domestic violence incidents where children are resident, and to inform them when there is a possibility that a child is in direct danger. In the event that the police are concerned about the child's or children's immediate safety, established child protection processes must be initiated.

> Each Domestic Violence Forum and ACPC [Area Child Protection Committee] should have clearly defined links, which should include cross-membership and identifying and working together on areas of common interest. The Domestic Violence Forum and ACPC should jointly contribute – in the context of the children's services plan – to an assessment of the incidence of children caught up in domestic violence, their needs, the adequacy of local arrangements to meet those needs, and the implications for local services.
>
> (Department of Health [DoH] 1999: 6.42)

Social services

> Normally, one serious incident or several lesser incidents of domestic violence where there is a child in the household would indicate that the social services department should carry out an initial assessment of the child and family, including consulting existing records.
>
> (Department of Health [DoH] 1999: 6.40)

The probation service

In 1998, the National Association of Probation Officers published a Domestic Violence Policy and Practice Guidance document. This document supplements an earlier position paper published by the Association of Chief Officers of Probation (ACOP) in 1996 which recommended that individual probation services adopt a policy on domestic violence which:

- confirmed that domestic violence should be treated as seriously as any other violent behaviour;
- endorsed the development of distinctive and effective community programmes for perpetrators;
- committed the service to working in a way which would promote the safety of survivors and children;
- emphasized the importance of working in partnership with other agencies; and
- acknowledged that the abuse of male power and control is a central feature to much domestic violence.

Moreover, Stelman *et al.* further note that the overall approach to practice has changed in recent years as probation officers acknowledge the importance of recognizing the impact of crimes on victims (1999: 228). In effect, this has changed the focus and methods of intervention generally and particularly with regards to the impact of domestic violence on women.

Where men might earlier have been placed on anger management programmes it is widely recognized that these programmes do not solve the problem of intimate violence and abuse. Countless men who abuse their female partners are not abusive in other settings, consequently intimate violence is not considered an extension of uncontrolled anger, and intervention strategies must reflect the fact that intimate abuse is about abusive power and control.

> Anger management programmes are predicated on the assumption that people who get angry do because they have lost control. Domestic violence perpetrators do not lose control. Their behaviour is, in fact, a series of methods of gaining control, and is itself very controlled as well as very controlling.
>
> (Stelman *et al.* 1999: 230)

A recommendation from the probation service is that the undergoing of perpetrator programmes should be mandatory for anyone convicted of a crime that included violence. This is particularly relevant to cases involving domestic abuse as the offence a man is convicted for is probably the last in a series of increasingly violent attacks on his female partner. However, there is a recommendation that women's support services and, when required, protection services need to be in place if the man responds violently. Recognizing that violent incidents usually escalate in frequency and severity should be taken into consideration by those deciding sentences and intervention strategies.

The Duluth model of intervention successfully used throughout the United States and more recently in the UK is covered in more detail in Chapter 10. Historically the probation service was not noted for success in inter-agency working; however, in recent years there has been a noticeable change in practice in many regions (Stelman *et al.* 1999: 232). In addition to working with the men, probation services often have a relationship with the wives and partners through the work done with families. Mullender (1996) emphasizes the need for staff at all levels in probation services, including those in administration, to be aware of a range of components related to domestic abuse. It is imperative that at no time is the man allowed to justify or excuse his behaviour in order to place the blame outside of his own personal responsibility. Staff need to be made aware of the need to adhere to established policies and procedures in place to ensure the security and safety of the woman and her family. This is especially relevant to confidential information and the necessity in some cases to keep the current location of the family secret. Mullender (1996) supports ACOP in advising departments, to provide a range of literature, including posters within the departments, for women who may be in abusive relationships. Information about abuse should be included as well as that about support groups, the local women's refuge, and help lines. Mullender further advocates that probation officers be adequately trained in benefits, housing, and legal matters in order that they can act in an advisory capacity, and in some instances, where appropriate, act as the woman's advocate.

Were probation services to become active members of local domestic violence forums, it would extend their knowledge and understanding of the wider concerns of women, in order that they are better placed to improve existing services. Probation officers are responsible for setting up and running perpetrator programmes, which to be successful need to incorporate the following principles.

PRINCIPLES OF GOOD PRACTICE FOR INTERVENTION PROGRAMMES

- Any programme should have the perspective of the woman at the forefront.
- Systems to protect the woman need to be in place before work on intervention with the man begins.
- The probation service ought to work in collaboration with other members of the multi-agency group to ensure the continuity of intervention. For example, were a further violent incident to occur the police would be required to notify the supervising probation officer.
- Any intervention is designed to ensure the man is required to challenge and take responsibility for his own violence. Some experts in the field believe that this can only be achieved if the perpetrator is required to undertake at least part of the intervention programmes within a group setting.
- Programmes should where possible be established within prisons and individuals convicted of any violent crime be required to attend as a condition of their sentence.
- The probation service should increase commitment to the support of the women and families of men convicted of violent crimes within intimate relationships.
- The primary measure of success of any intervention is directly related to a reduction in re-offending behaviour.

Local authorities

Following the publication of the Home Office document (1999) each local authority is required to set into place policies and procedures related to domestic violence that are understood and complied with by all its staff.

According to the Home Office (1999) a policy should:

- include details of good practice expected from all council staff;
- promote good practice in individual departments;
- provide a framework of co-ordinated and measurable responses to domestic violence by all key departments, including social services, education, housing, and youth and leisure services;
- include a clear emphasis on effective monitoring and evaluation;
- ensure that staff receive appropriate training.

Local authority social services departments

Domestic violence can be an important indicator of child abuse and vice versa: social workers should always look for one when the other is present, so that both abused adults and children can be made safe. In these cases, staff will need to be mindful that victims may be reluctant to disclose domestic violence where they have anxieties that social workers will be pre-occupied with child protection, or be judgmental.

(Home Office 1999)

The role of the social worker in child protection has been covered in more detail in Chapter 7, 'Domestic Violence and Children'.

The social worker's role in relation to children is carefully defined and documented within the DoH document from 1998, 'Inspection of Assessment, Planning and Decision-Making in Family Support Services. Classification: Children and Young People', reproduced in Appendix 4. There is a clear expectation that the various social service departments work collectively with the families of children in need of external support. Implicit in the role is the anticipation that whilst the needs of the family as a whole are supported the requirements of the child are paramount. In addition, where staff are working in close collaboration with other professionals and agencies, the social worker is required to operate within the statutory SSI framework.

In standard five, 'Inter-agency in Collaboration in Planning and Service Delivery', there is a stated expectation that the department ensures that there is a strategy for family support services as part of the children's service planning process. In addition, the services reflect the needs of children and families from a variety of ethnic and cultural backgrounds. The DoH document discusses 'SSD mechanisms designed to ensure each agency's family support work complements the others and avoids duplication of effort or resources [4.8]'.

In addition to being the major co-ordinators of child protection services, social workers are responsible for assessing the needs of other vulnerable groups within society. Therefore, the potential presence of domestic violence is also relevant to the responsibilities of social services departments in relation to older people and people with disabilities, drug and alcohol dependency and mental health problems.

The DoH for the past few years has been active in the areas of domestic abuse placing it high on the social justice agenda. The department appears committed to the development of practices and policies that provide that:

[a] holistic approach, including the provision of family support services and other measures to enable all the abused members of the family to make themselves safe may be a more effective intervention. This will include support, where appropriate, after the violence has ended, in terms of helping victims re-build their lives. Departments should also recognize that the involvement of domestic violence experts, such as experienced workers within the voluntary sector, can lead to better decision making. They can help ensure a comprehensive assessment of needs, risks, and protective steps, which can be taken.

(Home Office 1999)

It is now recognized that single disciplines and organizations have minimal impact on major areas of social concern unless they work co-operatively with other statutory and voluntary community groups and organizations.

Local authority education departments

As quoted earlier, Young *et al.* (2001: 4) recorded some disturbing information in the course of their research:

> Recent research on the understanding and attitudes to domestic violence of over 1,300 children aged 8–16 revealed disturbing statistics. Most children knew that domestic violence is common and considered fighting between parents to be wrong. However, over 75 per cent of 11–12 year old boys thought that women are hit if they make men angry. More boys than girls of all ages believed that some women deserve to be hit.
>
> (Young *et al.* 2001: 4)

It is recognized that domestic violence can and does affect children within the home even if there is no evidence of direct physical abuse. Schools, youth clubs, young persons associations, and children's organizations are all well placed to promote an understanding of the issues both to the children and to the staff. 'Teachers, auxiliary staff, educational welfare officers and others in regular contact with children and young people are well placed to notice whether a child might be affected by violence in the home' (Home Office 1999: 16). Organizations including WAFE provide a range of supportive literature for children and young people about domestic violence, on how they can receive help and how to keep themselves safe.

Victim Support Services

Victim Support Services (VSS) is an independent national charity funded in part by the Home Office to provide a comprehensive service to support victims of crime nationally. There are branches of the organization across the country. Each branch is staffed by a small number of permanent staff whilst the bulk of the work is done by trained volunteers. Clients are mainly referred by the police whilst an increasing number are referred by other organizations or are self-referred. The aim of the organization is to offer advice and practical support to any individual who has been the victim of a crime ranging from burglary or road traffic accidents to sexual offences and domestic violence. 'Victim Support also works for the rights of victims, witnesses and their families and greater awareness of the effects of crime' (Victim Support 2002: 5). VSS groups often complement the work of other agencies such as Women's Aid, whilst in recent years some local VSS organizations have taken over the role of supporting rape victims where no other local services exist. In relation to domestic violence, many local VSS organizations are representatives on multi-agency forums working with other agencies and individuals to support women who have been abused, throughout the survival process.

Whilst most of the clients have already reported the crime, an increasing number are self-referrals. This client group usually require support but do not wish to report the incident, and their wishes are respected throughout. The type and level of support is determined almost entirely by the needs of the client, although VSS emphasize that whilst they offer practical and emotional support they are not a counselling service. The woman (or man) in an abusive relationship is offered practical advice, including assistance to contact other helping agencies, and support through the criminal justice process and beyond if necessary. The nature of the relationship between the local police service and VSS is such that at the request of the victim, the volunteer assigned to the case can liaise directly with the police to clarify any queries the victim may have. In addition, the VSS operate the Victim Support's Witness Service, assisting victims, witnesses and their families and friends before, during and after a trial, a service that many individuals and families value highly. Like other agencies, VSS have an important role to play in the overall provision of services to enhance the care that is available to women and men who because of domestic violence have wide-ranging needs.

Health services and healthcare providers

As we have seen in previous chapters, each healthcare professional and organization has an important role to play in the recognition and assessment of abuse, planning and facilitating care for those being abused, and evaluating interventions. Within a multi-agency forum the emphasis should be to work with others to ensure that domestic violence is, and remains, high on the local and national social, political, legal and health agendas. Unfortunately, studies indicate that frequently healthcare professionals are absent from multi-agency forums, and consequently the level of intervention available in a healthcare setting is minimal.

To improve the status quo, health professionals should make an individual and collective commitment to improving the service currently offered to women in abusive relationships, especially in collaborative inter-agency ventures.

> Health authorities are under a statutory duty to improve the health of their populations and to do so in partnership with NHS agencies, local authorities and others, including the voluntary sector. The local Health Improvement Programme [HImP] sets out the strategic framework for achieving this and for modernising health services. Domestic violence as a key public health issue can be addressed within this HImP process.
>
> (Home Office 2002b)

National and local policy-makers

Since the late 1990s subsequent governments have placed women's issues generally, and violence against women specifically, on the national agenda. In particular a previous chapter addressed, in some depth, changes that were made in the law including Part IV of the Family Law Act 1997, and the Protection from Harassment Act 1997. In a Home Office publication *Living Without Fear* in 1999, the government spelled out its commitment to promoting a positive and pro-active approach to the prevention and management of violence within the home.

Readers should consider accessing the on-line resources available from the Department of Health, the Home Office, and the Office of the Deputy Prime Minister identified at the end of the book.

THE GOVERNMENT PERSPECTIVE: POLICY AND PROCESS

Policy-makers

As we have seen in previous chapters, many abused women experience special circumstances, which must be addressed by practitioners and policy-makers alike.

Among them are women with disabilities living in an abusive relationship, who may be prevented from leaving home as they are either excluded from refuges because of a lack of facilities, or there is insufficient alternative means of support. It is a well-known fact that overall, the needs of people with disabilities are not adequately provided for in many communities. This is often through lack of financial support, or staff shortages, limiting available alternatives. The 'care in the community' agenda is constantly compromised by underfunding, understaffing, and an over-reliance on home carers, many of whom are women. Consequently, the health and safety of vulnerable client groups, including those with mental illness, the aged, children, those with learning disabilities and the physically disabled, are already compromised through lack of adequate resources. Such situations are exacerbated when these individuals whose choices are already limited in the extreme, are within an abusive relationship, finding themselves with almost no choice other than to endure the abuse and violence.

It is crucial for policy-makers and practitioners at all levels to concede the impact and consequences of domestic violence, and ensure that alleviating it is a guiding principle when making and operationalizing health and social welfare policies.

CONCLUSION

> Virtually all local authorities had a domestic violence forum covering their area. However, evidence from the case studies suggested that the key local authority departments did not always attend regularly, or sent relatively junior members of staff, which affected the extent to which fora could influence policy.
>
> (Levison and Kenny 2002)

For multi-agency domestic violence forums to be successful, each individual agency needs to operate efficiently, effectively and with the needs of the women and children it seeks to serve at the forefront of any policies. Staff across the individual organization/agency require appropriate training and education that is regularly reviewed and updated. Wherever possible a named person, with expertise in the subject, should be appointed to take a lead role in policy development and practice. The individual (or team) requires sufficient authority, and access to the necessary funds to transform policy into practice both within the agency and within the forum. The final chapter explores a number of areas of practice across a variety of agencies that have succeeded in making a difference and may offer a way forward to better services for those involved in violence within the home.

Chapter 10

Existing challenges and future opportunities

CHALLENGING EXISTING PRACTICE

There has been a significant growth in the number of healthcare initiatives across the United Kingdom specifically designed to improve practice related to the identification and management of domestic abuse in a variety of health and social care settings. This chapter summarizes obstacles that may inhibit good practice development by identifying the challenges currently facing practitioners.

MAINTAINING THE SILENCE IN HEALTHCARE SETTINGS

Throughout, this book has explored the various reasons why staff may not respond to the needs of clients within a domestic abuse situation in a way that is either pro-active or effective. Such reasons include:

- Even when victims are identified, doctors' and nurses' attitudes are ambivalent about the nature of domestic abuse, with many believing that it is not their business to intervene.
- Some staff continue to consider domestic abuse as a private matter and therefore unless the woman directly asks for help believe that it is not their business.
- Occasionally staff exhibit inappropriate behaviour that discourages clients from disclosing the abuse or their fear of it. Staff may ignore signs that abuse is taking place and on occasion may avoid spending time with the client/patient.
- Repeatedly, studies indicate that there is inadequate education and training at all levels of each organization.
- Research in the subject area needed to effectively guide policy-making is often inconclusive, which leads some organizations to ignore the issues or to offer minimum levels of care.
- It is necessary for some professionals to create psychological distance from the problem, often because the subject is 'too close to home'. Organizations without supportive domestic violence policies for the well-being of staff may have little success implementing wider initiatives for client groups.
- A lack of understanding of the abusive process may lead to the frustration of health professionals when victims return repeatedly to a violent situation but continue to

revisit healthcare settings for support. This frustration may be exhibited to the client in negative ways thus making it problematical for the client in the future.

- Too many health organizations omit to design policies and protocols that guide and enhance relevant practice. Therefore, staff are left uncertain as to their responsibilities or appropriate courses of action.
- Whilst there are many successful inter-agency forums operating across the country the evidence indicates that recurrently healthcare representation is absent, perhaps reflecting the ambiguous position of health in such initiatives.

Therefore, local policy-making and staff development initiatives ought to commence by challenging existing beliefs and behaviours within the organization, build on good practice and facilitate attitude change through education. Furthermore, senior management teams have to be challenged as to how they intend to support and provide practical assistance to their own employees living in domestic violence situations.

Davina James-Hanman (1998), talking of collaborative inter-agency, inter-professional co-operation, states that:

> We have to work together to address this issue and indeed, in many areas, enormous changes have taken place over the last decade. Sadly, though, of all of the public-funded agencies which have a role to play, it is the health service, excepting a few isolated pockets of good practice, which has been one of the slowest to respond.

James-Hanman acknowledged at the time of writing that in the preceding two years significant national and local initiatives related to domestic violence in healthcare had begun to make an impact on the hitherto relatively poor service for abused women. She cited Sheila Adams, the Deputy Director of the Health Services, who previously identified the barriers to change in this area as:

- The fact that the health service is accident-focused rather than injury-focused means that health interventions repeatedly deal with consequences rather than causes, especially in the realms of domestic abuse.
- A national deficit in healthcare staff training and education has resulted in few of them being in a position to understand the dynamics of domestic abuse or the health consequences, therefore staff do not know what to do (practically).
- Staff may be embarrassed to ask the question, or fail to do so because they do not want to get 'involved'. In addition, studies have identified that a common reason for non-intervention is the fear of unsettling the client/patient relationship.
- Untrained staff regularly possess misconceptions about domestic violence; many assume domestic violence only happens to women from low social classes with low self-esteem and poor education. Thus, staff remain oblivious to the needs of many individuals within abusive intimate relationships.
- Studies reveal that healthcare staff either through a lack of understanding or because they feel unable to make a difference, have expressed feelings of powerlessness when dealing with clients who have been abused.
- Other staff use the excuse of insufficient time to spend dealing with a woman in an abusive situation.

Indeed, to a point, the last reason may be true as the facilitation process can be exceptionally time-consuming, involving many other agencies and professionals. However, healthcare professionals should remember that the client requires time, understanding and compassion but most importantly the opportunity to make her own informed choices. Or perhaps staff view 'time spent' as 'time wasted' if the woman returns to her partner only to present back in the department at a later date. Research in many disciplines has identified the frustrations professionals experience when the client fails to take what to them seems to be sound advice.

Domestic violence is an emotive subject; one that historically individuals and organizations alike have failed to address. The reasons for this have been explored in depth in earlier chapters, what we have to do now is move the discussion forward and identify affirmative actions for future practice. There exists a plethora of literature related to the management of change both for individuals and for organizations generally; therefore, this section focuses specifically on overcoming barriers to implementing change in the area of domestic violence practice.

Key points

Additional barriers to change include:

- Staff resistance: domestic violence is still viewed by many as a 'personal' problem rather than a social one. All too often domestic abuse is identified as a 'private family matter', or excepted as a 'cultural norm'.
- Too many individuals including healthcare practitioners dealing with the aftermath of an assault or other effects of the abuse, may have their own personal issues to deal with.
- Various studies indicate that at present innumerable healthcare professionals remain untrained in the recognition and management of domestic abuse and violence. Therefore, either they are professionally unaware, or, if they are aware, they do not have the knowledge and skills to manage it effectively.
- Healthcare organizations currently operate in a milieu that demands staff perform to changing government priorities, with numerous national and local targets. Therefore, the traditional role of healthcare practitioners is regularly transformed to meet these often-competing needs. Hence, staff training may focus on the attainment of current government-led clinical targets with domestic violence falling off the agenda.
- For organizational change to be effective usually there has to be a named staff member to take the initiative forward. According to James-Hanman (1998), a lack of a national policy framework and/or a lack of a nominated officer at corporate level within trusts often inhibits organizational change.
- Similarly, studies have established that failure to provide a named representative, with sufficient power to facilitate change within an agency or organization, to act for the agency or organization on local and national domestic violence forums, inhibits major change.

COMMITMENT AT A NATIONAL LEVEL

Whilst some progress has been made in placing domestic violence on the national agenda it is only recently that the significant work of the women's movements and other organizations has been overtly recognized by the government. Currently the Department of Health and the Home Office in conjunction with other government departments have published widely a set of papers related to the recognition and management of domestic abuse. The primary message contained within these documents is that domestic violence and abuse are not to be tolerated under any circumstances. Furthermore, local agencies and organizations, including the criminal justice services, health services, local authorities and, among them, social services, have a statutory responsibility to work collectively and individually on behalf of the abused person in the development of wide-ranging effective strategies, policies and protocols.

LOCAL POLICIES

The Women's Aid Federation for England (2001) 'Guidelines to Good Practice' authored by Dr Humphreys are reproduced (with permission) in full in Appendix 2, and are explored below.

Principles to underpin domestic violence policies

Local domestic violence forums, provided that they work together for common aims, have the ability to enable complementary interventions to be established across a range of services. The following principles, collated from a variety of sources, should underpin individual and collective initiatives.

1   The safety of the woman and any child or children and others have to be paramount at all times. The first priority of intervention is to establish and implement policies and protocols that protect the victim from further harm.
2   All policies and procedural guidelines require regular review by members of the communities not represented by the majority culture (e.g., communities of colour, the gay/lesbian/bisexual community, people who are on low incomes) (the Domestic Abuse Intervention Project [DAIP] 2000).
3   All practices and policies should be continually evaluated and discussed to ensure their effectiveness in protecting all victims.
4   Intervention strategies must reflect a staff–client model of intervention, founded on client empowerment.
5   Large organizations ought to consider appointing at least one senior staff member to initiate and provide a service to educate and train staff and to establish local policy groups.
6   Organization policy groups are tasked with devising intervention strategies that emerge from the on-going work of multi-agency forums.
7   Initial and on-going training has to be available for continuous staff training and development.

8   All interventions must take account of the power imbalance between the assailant and the victim, and the professional and the victim.

Designing local health organization policies

Having identified the essential overarching principles for effective policy-making and implementation, staff need to address the standards required for specific policies.

An organization has to ensure that:

1   Staff and patients/clients recognize and agree that domestic abuse is unacceptable and that every effort is made to support those enduring abuse within the home.
2   The safety of the client, the client's family and the staff is paramount.
3   Staff have adequate support in the form of clinical supervision or similar, to enable them to maintain their own psychological health if called upon to deal with an abused client/patient.
4   Attention is given to diversity and equality issues.
5   Women's Aid identifies a requirement to set protocols to meet the specific needs of children and families, vulnerable adults, community care recipients and perpetrators; practice guidelines for front-line workers; safety policies for workers; and policies specific to the service provided by each department and organization.
6   In addition, any organization is obliged to 'embed policies within the organization, through training, guidance, the development of appropriate procedures and service provision' (WAFE 2003).
7   Detailed guidelines, which explicate the issues for practice and are developed where possible in conjunction with prospective client user groups, should be provided.

COLLECTING DATA

One criticism of current intervention models is that repeatedly there is an inconsistency related to data collection. The terms 'domestic violence' and 'abuse' are generic terms that often have no shared meaning between agencies and organizations. As data-recording is usually influenced by the definition of the phenomena being explored, it is unsurprising if research in the field subsequently demonstrates inconsistency. Consequently, the many 'hidden' aspects of domestic abuse such as sexual, emotional, financial and psychological abuse, and including the effects on the children, are inadequately reported. For these aspects to be reported they first have to be acknowledged and included within any assessment documentation.

Humphreys et al. (2001) advocate for a system of monitoring that enhances disclosure and has shared meaning within the multi-agency partnership. In addition, they advocate for clear lines of responsibility for collating data and referrals within each agency to ensure a systematic and co-ordinated approach to intervention. Only when these structures are in place is a clear picture of the nature and size of domestic abuse in any one locality possible. Once the data are established then the professionals have a powerful argument for increased or additional resources both locally and nationally. 'Good practice is indicated where attention has been paid to the broad scope of policy development and where there is clarity about referral and procedures' (Humphreys et al. 2000: 5).

Some organizations, for instance, the police and in some areas of healthcare practice, are appointing staff with a specific remit to act in cases of domestic abuse. The function within the designated role may include staff development, policy-making, inter-agency collaboration and co-operation as well as direct client intervention.

ESTABLISHED PROJECTS: AN OVERVIEW

There have been many successful intervention programmes in the last decade and this section briefly explores some of the well-known ones.

The Domestic Abuse Intervention Project (DAIP) in Duluth, Minnesota

The Domestic Abuse Intervention Project (DAIP) in Duluth, Minnesota, now known world-wide as the Duluth Model, is arguably the most well-known multi-agency approach to understanding and managing domestic violence and abuse in existence. DAIP is a comprehensive community-based programme for intervention in domestic abuse cases. Its primary aim is to co-ordinate the response of the many agencies and practitioners who respond to domestic violence cases across a specific community.

> The project involves community organizing and advocacy that examines training programs, policies, procedures and texts – intake forms, report formats, assessments, evaluations, checklists and other materials. We ask, how does each practice, procedure, form or brochure either enhance or compromise victim safety?
>
> (Domestic Abuse Intervention Project 2000)

The programme is based on the premise that a shared approach to intervention over a range of services improves the chances of survival from harm for the woman and her child or children. Multi-agency forums operating under the principles devised by DAIP work towards negotiating common understandings among themselves in order to minimize the negative impact of fragmented philosophies and responses on the victims of domestic violence. 'These understandings make central the victim's experience of violence and coercion and ongoing threats to her safety' (Domestic Abuse Intervention Project 2000). DAIP believes that safe and effective practices in the field of domestic abuse can be achieved when the following principles are adopted by a multi-agency forum.

Guiding principles of Intervention

1 Whenever possible, the burden of confronting abusers and placing restrictions on their behaviours should rest with the community, not the victim.
2 To make fundamental changes in a community's response to violence against women, individual practitioners must work co-operatively, guided by training, job descriptions, and standardized practices that are all oriented toward the desired changes.
3 Intervention must be responsive to the totality of harm done by the violence rather than be incident- or punishment-focused.
4 Protection of the victim must take priority when two intervention goals clash.

5 Intervention practices must reflect a basic understanding of and a commitment to accountability to the victim, whose life is most impacted by our individual and collective actions.

Adherence to these principles helps to produce consistent results regardless of the beliefs or values of an individual practitioner. They are reproduced with permission from the Domestic Abuse Intervention Project (DAIP) in Duluth, Minnesota.

Many individual projects in healthcare, police work, the probation services and social services in the UK are based on principles established within the Duluth model of intervention.

Domestic Violence Matters (DVM project Islington)

'The project was an innovative response to domestic violence in Islington. It aimed to provide a civilian crisis intervention service, to follow up police responses, enhance law enforcement responses and create consistent and co-ordinated responses among local agencies' (Kelly *et al.* 1999). This project, established in 1993, utilized civilian people to act as support workers, providing an out-of-hours support system for women that had been involved in a domestic abuse incident. The project originally set out to determine whether, and how, immediate and on-going civilian support could improve the service offered to abused women. Over the three years, DVM worked with 1,236 individuals, in relation to 1,542 incidents, and found that over two-thirds of referrals to DVM were received outside normal office hours. The statistics showed that:

- 99 per cent of service users were female
- 99 per cent of perpetrators were male
- 21 per cent of the women were black.
- ten per cent were from other ethnic minorities
- five per cent were disabled.

The overall project was deemed successful in that it offered a rapid response to an incident by trained individuals offering both support, and where necessary the ability to act as an advocate for the woman. The scheme was generally acknowledged to have a positive effect given an interventionist pro-active approach that led to a more co-ordinated response from the various agencies. This programme has subsequently been used as a model of good practice by other districts and counties (Kelly *et al.* 1999).

Other projects

Key point

Readers are recommended to the *Domestic Violence & Health Practice Directory* (2000) reproduced on the Women's Aid web site. This offers a comprehensive list of recent initiatives in a range of healthcare settings across the country. In addition the reader is directed to the set of briefing notes: 'Reducing Domestic Violence . . . What Works' published by the Policing and Reducing Crime Unit within the Home Office (2000) that have been referred to throughout previous chapters.

Several projects focus on the detection and intervention of abuse during pregnancy, including the Leeds Inter-Agency Project: Health and Social Care Project.

> Partnership work has led to the development of a mandatory training programme for all midwives, consisting of a half-day session, three-month reflective practice period with the submission of a piece of written work, and a full-day session.

At the time of reporting (Women's Aid 2003), over 270 midwives had completed or were currently undertaking the programme accredited for Post Registration Education and Practice (PREP).

The Leeds project is one of the most extensive in the country and has been subsequently extended to include sessions into an on-going programme for obstetricians and gynae-cologists, and the development of a specific training programme for administrative and ancillary staff. The project continued by establishing a steering group to develop a pro-gramme that included staff training and support, development of guidelines and a protocol for screening, monitoring and auditing service delivery and partnership working. The initiative was further expanded to include training and development for nursing and medical staff within the Accident and Emergency department, with the intention of further expansion across all the trust's areas.

The Leeds Inter-Agency Project: Health and Social Care Project also carried out a number of other initiatives of note including:

- work with disabled women
- work with children and young people
- work with social services and probation services.

Routine screening

Mezey et al. (2001) reporting on a study for routine screening of pregnant women high-lighted that although domestic violence screening may become routine, it should never be dealt with by a simple 'tick box' exercise. The study illustrated that whilst a significant number of the women accepted screening to be reasonable practice they qualified their responses by indicating that although asking about domestic violence was, in theory, acceptable to women, the health professional had to be perceived as caring, sympathetic and interested in their response. They needed to be able to provide the time to listen, they needed to be perceived as competent, in terms of being able to provide relevant infor-mation about sources of help and support, and they needed to be able to offer private confidential time (a rarity in maternity services) (Mezey et al. 2001). The authors of the study concluded that for routine screening to be successful, given the existing pressures on clinical staff in maternity services, then consideration should be given to the appoint-ment of specialist domestic violence workers to co-ordinate training and support staff in this work.

Other projects have focused on the development of local protocols including the design and distribution of a range of literature made readily available in healthcare settings. Several projects have explored the use of assessment tools including body maps and photo-graphic evidence to enhance future successful prosecution, whilst others have investigated the use of standardized screening questionnaires.

More than a few of the identified projects have been connected to multi-agency initiatives whilst others have focused more specifically on the design of training materials. Camden and Islington Domestic Violence Forum was one of the first to write a training pack for use by a range of agencies but with specific information for healthcare providers. More recently, the Department of Health commissioned a manual for healthcare workers, which is available for downloading from the DoH web site. The manual is useful for individuals wishing to enhance their own knowledge, or as a basis for staff development across departments.

Wakefield District Primary Care Domestic Violence Project is a project intended to bring together health services, voluntary and community sectors and a range of criminal justice agencies with the aim of improving the well-being of women and their children and assisting them to live healthy lives free from violence and abuse. The programme was established in 2000 and evaluation is on-going. Various community projects, and especially inter-agency models of practice have emerged as a direct result of the successful work undertaken in Duluth, Minnesota.

According to Hester *et al.* (2000), violence prevention for school pupils and young people is still under-developed in the UK. However, there are now curriculum materials available for both primary and secondary schools. It is anticipated that if children and young people are allowed to explore the notion of violence, especially that which occurs within relationships and in the home, it may influence their attitudes and thus behaviours as they grow into adulthood. Hester *et al.* (2000) identified how some domestic violence forums have produced plays and workshops for schools and youth groups and noted the work of the Violence Free Relationship Programme, co-ordinated by the Sandwell against Domestic Violence Project. The aim of the project is:

> to provide students with an opportunity to explore attitudes and beliefs that may contribute to the manifestation of abuse in a relationship. It also encourages young people to explore and develop strategies to avoid or address abusive relationships and has been identified as an example of good practice.
>
> (Hester *et al.* 2000: 2)

The number of projects in various aspects of domestic abuse is growing almost daily. Readers wishing to keep abreast of developments are advised to utilize the web addresses and contact addresses found within the appendices. Some organizations undertake excellent work related to specific minority groups; for example, women who have specific needs as a result of a disability, their sexual orientation, their immigration status or their ethnic or religious background. Increased interest in various aspects of the phenomena including domestic violence within the workplace, amongst refugees, against men and lesbian women, means that the literature is rapidly expanding.

Intervention programmes for men

At the time of writing, Mullender and Burton (2000) estimated that there were up to 30 perpetrator programmes operating in the UK. It is their belief that for any perpetrator programme to be successful, the man first has to accept responsibility for the violence and abuse recognizing that he is required to change both his attitude and his behaviours. The most common model is one based on a cognitive-behavioural or psycho-educational approach. The model recognizes that abusive and violent behaviour is learned behaviour and that with a great deal of work, it can be unlearned. In addition, programmes are designed to challenge the men's belief systems that convince them that they have a right to control women in intimate relationships. The programmes aim to 'foster mutual respect' and each of them requires men 'to accept responsibility for their past actions and future choices'. It will require, too, 'regular group attendance', will 'challenge denial and minimalization, and harness the dynamic of the group to do the same' (Mullender and Burton 2000: 1).

It is now generally accepted by those working in the field of domestic abuse, that other approaches such as anger management, substance misuse programmes, couple counselling or family counselling undertaken as stand-alone programmes have little, if any, positive effects, and in some instances might prove dangerous to the woman and her children. Where in the past anger management, for example, has been viewed as a positive intervention the argument against is that the man already manages his anger, he actively targets his female partner and uses the anger as a deliberate means of coercion and control. Nevertheless, where alcohol or substance misuse is present, parallel interventions may assist in the overall success.

Criticism has also been levelled at counselling programmes designed to support the woman by attempting to raise her self-esteem, arguing that this puts the onus on the woman rather than locating the violence with the abusive man. However, where women express a need for this type of support it ought to be made available. Often women find that the mutual support available through women's groups is a powerful means of dealing with their personal challenges.

An evaluative project on male perpetrator programmes in Scotland, undertaken by Dobash et al. (1996: 1), concluded that: 'The research suggests that criminal justice based programmes using cognitive behavioural principles may make a positive contribution towards a reduction in violence against women in the home.'

However, Mullender and Burton (2000) have expressed concern at

- the number of men enrolled on programmes who failed to show;
- the rate of drop out from programmes;
- the lack of long-term evaluative studies so that one could not predict with any certainty longer-term successes; and
- the number of cases where the woman was not apprised of the perpetrator's progress, or even if he had dropped out of the programme. There was concern that failure to inform the woman might put her at increased risk.

Dobash et al. (2000) describe the dual model of intervention as a pro-feminist approach designed to enable men to gain insight into their own behaviour and emotions in order that they might end their violent and abusive behaviours.

Established programmes of note, for male perpetrators, include, according to Dobash et al. (1996: 1), CHANGE and the LDVPP projects established in Scotland. They are both criminal justice-based programmes designed to re-educate men who have been found guilty of offences involving violence against their partner. Men participate in the programme as a condition of a probation order. The programmes offer 'structured, "challenging" group work, conducted on a weekly basis for six to seven months, with the men required to attend as a condition of sentencing'.

These and other international perpetrator programmes have often emerged as a result of the work undertaken in Duluth, Minnesota. The power and control wheels, as discussed in Chapter 2, emerged from the countless discussions, held over a long period of time, by numerous women as to what constitutes abusive behaviour and what women defined as acceptable behaviour. Experts believe that only when men through intensive group work, recognize, accept, take responsibility for, and challenge the behaviours identified in the first wheel is it possible for them to move towards the behaviours identified in the second wheel.

Increasingly in the UK as part of a rehabilitative approach the undertaking of a perpetrator programme is becoming a requirement of sentencing. Where previously men may have been encouraged or required to attend anger control and management sessions these, according to Mullender (1996: 213), are no longer viewed as appropriate methods for dealing with abusive men as 'these men are fully in control of the victim they target . . . and their so-called "anger" is actually a need to dominate and control'.

The Domestic Violence Intervention Project (DVIP), undertaken in London, combines a Violence Prevention Project (VPP) that works with men to challenge and change their abusive behaviour, with a simultaneously offered Women's Support Service (WSS) to work with partners of men on VPP and women who self-refer. The overall philosophy is to empower women and increase their safety, and to stop men's use of violence and abuse. In a two-year evaluation of the DVIP by the Joseph Rowntree Foundation:

> The researchers conclude that programmes for violent men when combined with proactive responses to women have a part in co-ordinated responses to domestic violence. However, work with men should not be undertaken without an attached support service for women, and there should be routes onto programmes for voluntarily referred men.

> (Joseph Rowntree Foundation 1998: 4)

The London Probation Association announced in 2002 that it was their intention to expand a project based on the Duluth model of intervention across a number of boroughs in London. The aims of the project, designed to improve the response to victims and intervention for perpetrators, include:

- creating an approach focusing on victim safety;
- developing 'best practice' policies and protocols that are part of an integrated response to domestic violence;
- ensuring a supportive community infrastructure for victims;
- providing both sanctions and rehabilitation opportunities for perpetrators;
- reducing the harm that domestic violence does to children;
- evaluating the co-ordinated community response from the standpoint of victim safety.

The National Association for Domestic Violence Perpetrator Programmes and Associated Support (2000) published a comprehensive set of standards developed from the Statement of Principles of the National Practitioners' Association. The standards are used by practitioners across the country dealing with male perpetrators.

COMMENTS ON INTERVENTIONS TO DATE

Jukes (2002: 324) noted that where interventions are focused at the wider social risk factors such as poverty or alcohol consumption, subsequent research rarely evaluated the projects in terms of domestic violence reduction.

> Although interventions that alter the prevalence of any of these risk factors may alter the prevalence of domestic violence, few programmes that seek primarily to reduce, for example, poverty or consumption of alcohol evaluate the impact on the prevalence of domestic violence.

A review of international literature on successful interventions concludes that a single approach is rarely successful. Not surprisingly, Jukes (2002) argues that training alone has limited outcomes unless it is accompanied by local media campaigns, literature, and readily available support from various agencies. Kelly and Humphreys (2000) found that although 24-hour help lines run by organizations such as Women's Aid, Refuge, Victim supportline and Childline, as well as those run by local groups, have proved to be very successful as outreach initiatives, funding for such endeavours remains problematic. Other help lines run by local community groups, or the specialist help lines for women from ethnic minority origins, report comparable successes and face similar financial challenges.

FUTURE PROJECTS

In October 2002, the government (Ukon-line.gov) announced plans to carry out a range of studies to establish the economic and social costs of domestic violence against women. The aims of the study are to estimate the costs to organizations that deal with the aftermath of domestic abuse including the criminal justice system departments such as the police, the court costs and the lost working days. The project team also plan to investigate longer-term expenses incurred through prolonged ill-health, reduced productivity in the workplace, and the on-going need for family intervention as a result of having been in an abusive relationship. It is anticipated that the 'study will also begin to unravel how the economic burden of domestic violence falls on individual women and their families. It will start to assess the price women pay for losing their homes and living with emotional and psychological distress, for example' (Ukon-line.gov 2002).

With the current high profile of domestic abuse and violence it is predicted that a continuing growth in projects for the foreseeable future is to be expected. However, interventions are costly and the replication of existing projects or the design of new ones without a more co-ordinated and systematic national approach is arguably an inappropriate use of scarce resources.

Key points

New research needs to build on what is already known, utilize existing expertise especially from women survivors and women's groups, and include studies that relate to the wider social, political and public organizational systems, structures and philosophies.

In March 2003 WAFE, in partnership with British Telecom, published a guide to employers on protocols to support staff in the workplace. Many public sector organizations, especially those in the healthcare services, have significant numbers of female staff, and yet few, if any, of those organizations have policies to support those staff who are being abused at home. Now is the time for senior healthcare management to put domestic abuse on its own organization's agenda, accepting that staff can only improve client care related to domestic abuse situations when they themselves feel valued and safe.

Chapter 11

Making a difference – the way forward

This chapter refers directly to the health needs of abused women; however, the same principles should be applied to those individuals in abusive relationships who are male, gay, bisexual or transgender clients. The chapter explores how domestic abuse can be challenged by those working in healthcare arenas through established good practice including aspects of multi-disciplinary intervention as appropriate.

PREVENTION OF VIOLENCE TO WOMEN

> Prevention of domestic violence to women can be conceptualised in two ways: preventing violence occurring in the first place, or, more commonly, preventing repeat attacks. The vast bulk of work world-wide has focused on attempting to reduce the incidence of repeat victimisation by provision of legal, welfare and social supports for women; and to a more limited extent attempting to control and change male offenders.
>
> (Morley and Mullender 1994: 16)

The report suggests that early intervention in the violent process is an essential factor if the man is to change his abusive behaviour. It is extensively documented that over time domestic abuse and violence escalate in both frequency and severity and that the longer it goes unchallenged by the perpetrator the worse it becomes. Moreover, his violence is almost certainly sustained across future sexual relationships thus endangering the well-being of every woman with whom he has a relationship.

SEEKING HELP

For intervention to be effective women need to be convinced that seeking help at the earliest opportunity is the preferred strategy for survival. Regrettably the majority of international prevalence studies indicate that a woman is injured multiple times before she seeks professional help, whilst others are mortally wounded.

Therefore, the persistence of domestic violence and abuse ought to be challenged by those who are in a position to do so. Only when the topic is placed high on the health and social care agenda at all levels of practice can those being abused have a voice that is heard.

Dynamics of the relationship between the client and the professional

> And what is worse is the expectation by those agencies that do offer help that women should behave in a certain way; that they should, if they want to get sympathy and understanding behave like a 'proper victim'.
>
> (James-Hanman 1998: 405)

Repeatedly when organizational or departmental policy is established, the woman's (abused person's) voice is silent either because her views are not sought or because once given they are frequently moderated by the 'expert'. Whilst the 'professional' has access to the research and readings on domestic abuse giving them a wider perspective, the woman being abused has 'expert' knowledge of a man's violence. At the point a woman seeks healthcare intervention, she conceivably possesses sophisticated survival skills and thus is well placed to predict his response to any outside intervention.

Arguably, the key to 'successful' intervention is for the healthcare provider to accept that the violence is probably entrenched and that the woman has complex reasons for staying. Therefore any solution is equally complex and may even mean that the woman chooses to stay in the relationship; what the healthcare professional can do is offer her alternatives and respect the choices she makes.

Listening skills

> So learning how to listen to women, how to validate their experiences and give them a safe space in which to make choices is one of the most important services we can offer.
>
> (James-Hanman 1998: 407)

Key point

- Any offer of assistance should acknowledge the right of the woman to choose for herself the next step to take.
- Never underestimate the danger she says she is in.
- Never underestimate her ability to find and utilize her own coping strategies.
- Support should be unconditional and non-judgemental, even if this is the third or fourth time of her seeking it.
- In no way should the woman be made to feel that she is to blame for what has happened to her.
- Never forget that 'women are entitled to the guarantee, protection and enjoyment of all their human rights, and that violence against women is a fundamental violation of those rights and their dignity' (James-Hanman 1998: 407).

In addition, healthcare staff in all settings need to be alert to the following:

- Expect to have contact with women experiencing domestic violence.
- Recognize that on occasions the abuse can be female on male, or occur within same sex-relationships, and may affect transgender individuals.
- Understand the dynamics of domestic abuse and its impact on the woman and her children specifically and the family as a whole.
- Be aware of the specific needs of minority groups including those women with disabilities, or from minority ethnic backgrounds, and those women for whom English is not their first language.

Providing a safe environment

Safety planning according to Humphreys *et al.* (2001: 6) has to be the primary concern of everyone in the organization both for the safety of the client and her children but also, equally important, for the safety of staff. The concept of risk and risk assessment is covered in detail later in the chapter. Humphreys emphasizes that

> At an organizational level, safety planning needs to include a range of measures including safe premises and access, information for service users, and confidentiality, including not passing on information about abused women and children to others, particularly violent partners or their associates.
>
> (Humphreys *et al.* 2001, web site)

It is essential that if abuse is suspected, where possible the healthcare professional provides an opportunity for the client to speak privately to a member of staff, preferably one trained to deal with domestic abuse. Previous chapters have highlighted the necessity for independent interpreters wherever possible, for women for whom English is not their first language. Women with learning difficulties, or mental health problems, may require the support of an independent advocate with the requisite specialist understanding of the client's needs.

Conducting an interview with a client in an abusive relationship can be distressing for all parties. Historically the role of many healthcare professionals has been one of 'diagnosing the problem', finding solutions and offering treatments. However, domestic abuse is one of those circumstances where outcomes are rarely so clear-cut, where the process can be lengthy and during it, the woman may consult with a range of health and social care agencies. If the client is ever to reach an acceptable solution, each consultation ought to result in her feeling respected and empowered.

Any interviews with the client should be unhurried, she should feel as comfortable as possible in the circumstances. As well, it is important that her views are accepted as valid and that she feels safe.

Supporting a client who is in an abusive relationship: DO's and DON'Ts

Do

- Give priority to her safety – explore ways of maximizing her safety whether she decides to leave her partner or not.
- Take her seriously, believe what she tells you.
- Respond positively, give her your support.
- Take her fears seriously, her life may be in danger.
- Tell her the violence is not her fault.
- Let her know she is not alone, tell her she can always see you again.
- Find out what she wants to do and help her achieve it.
- Bear in mind that she may have been exposed to racism, language, and cultural barriers.
- Respect her wishes and accept her decisions.
- Explore the options with her and talk through with her how she can avoid being abused.
- Keep in contact if possible.

Don't

- Don't tell her what she should do next.
- Don't try solving all her problems – the decisions are hers.
- Don't pressurize her into agreeing to action with which she is uncomfortable.
- Don't make choices for her.
- Don't be judgemental of her actions and choices.
- Don't be sceptical or fob her off when she comes to you for help.
- Don't ask her what she did to provoke the violence.
- Don't give up on her, just because things are taking longer than you think that they should or if she hasn't taken your advice or because she has gone back to her partner.
- Don't promise to pass messages or facilitate contact with the partner in any way, as this may endanger both you and the woman.
- Don't give *anyone* the address or telephone number of where she is staying. This includes other professionals, unless there is a very strong over-riding reason for them to know, such as child protection, as abusers often persuade others to make enquiries on their behalf. Where there are child protection concerns, establish the identity of the professional you are passing the information on to and ensure that the number you are telephoning is the correct office number for the department they claim to represent.
- Don't set pre-conditions for supporting her, such as that she must prosecute him, obtain an injunction or leave him.
- Don't withdraw your support if she decides to stay in the relationship. Indeed, this situation may require more support rather than less.

Reproduced with permission of Newham Domestic Violence Forum
(Domestic Violence Directory, section two, p. 2)

Collecting data

Earlier chapters explored the challenge of collecting appropriate data in healthcare settings. What the professional must consider when determining what information is required partly depends upon her or his understanding of domestic abuse.

In the first instance, the healthcare professional requires information that enables an appropriate client assessment to be made in order that effective short-, medium- and, if required, long-term intervention is agreed. Information also needs to be recorded by staff in a detailed and systematic form, as it may be required later in civil or criminal proceedings. Where information is of a particularly sensitive nature, it may be necessary to provide secure storage; this is especially important if a risk assessment is undertaken and the findings shared amongst professional groups. Agreement about the nature of the data to be collected, its storage, the rules of confidentiality, methods of analysis and who collects it, should be in place once a local multi-agency forum is established. It is then viable to collate statistics in a meaningful way in order to respond to local needs and improve local provision, moreover results can be utilized to inform the national agenda. With careful consideration and forethought and with a uniform approach to data collection across agencies, it is feasible for comparisons between provisions to be undertaken.

Confidentiality

Issues related to confidentiality have been explored throughout. The issues are two-fold. First, staff have to consider the implications of sharing confidential information across departments, and with other agencies. Generally, the rule is that the client's permission is sought before information is shared. However, in cases with a potential risk to children this condition may have to be waived. Where the client is seriously injured and thus a crime has been committed, with the police services involved confidentiality may be compromised. The subject of confidentiality requires careful consideration within departments including Accident and Emergency, where comprehensive policy guidelines need establishing.

The second major consideration is ensuring that clinical records with personal information, including the client's whereabouts, are kept in a safe place. If the client chooses to leave the relationship and seeks refuge, it is essential that the abuser is not able to gain access to this information. All staff should be made aware of the possible consequences of inadvertently disclosing information in all domestic violence cases. This is particularly pertinent within obstetric care where the mother keeps her notes and the partner is often in attendance at ante-natal visits. Protocols for recording sensitive information are devised to ensure staff are aware of the status quo and to facilitate continuity of care, but also as a means of recording injuries evidence of which might be required at a later date.

Screening women

The question of routine screening has been debated within previous chapters, and the consensus is that women are generally not averse to being asked by the healthcare practitioner about domestic abuse. However, a study undertaken by Richardson and others, within a GP primary care setting in Hackney, and published in 2002, found that whilst:

- over a third of women attending general practices had experienced physical violence from a male partner or former partner;
- most women who had experienced physical violence were not identified by general practitioners, according to data extracted from their medical records; and
- women pregnant in the previous year were at high risk for current physical violence;

nevertheless, 'A substantial minority of women object to routine questioning about domestic violence'. This led the research team to conclude that: 'With the high prevalence of domestic violence, health professionals should maintain a high level of awareness of the possibility of domestic violence, especially affecting pregnant women, but the case for screening is not yet convincing' (Richardson *et al.* 2002: 274). Accordingly, when designing operational policies and procedures healthcare staff need to consider whether to undertake routine screening. For example, where there is visible evidence of an injury probably caused by domestic abuse, this cannot be ignored. Neither should a healthcare professional avoid asking questions if in the course of the assessment process, or on-going care process, she or he has reason to believe that the client is in an abusive relationship. The professional code of conduct and professional guidelines of healthcare practitioners are unanimous in the belief that staff have a duty of care to clients, and that ignoring the facts might in certain circumstances be construed as negligence.

Providing information to the client

Studies have shown that some women remain in abusive relationships because they are unaware that viable alternatives exist. If one agrees that knowledge equates to power then, by providing adequate information, healthcare practitioners are able to make a difference to some of the abused women they encounter. However, where the client is accompanied to the department, the clinic, or the unit by their partner, it is perhaps inappropriate to offer written materials on domestic abuse. The Women's Aid Federation and some local police services, or multi-agency forums, provide small cards with emergency help-line numbers, available for purchase by healthcare organizations. If issued to women they are small enough to hide away in a purse, reducing the risk of discovery by the partner. Information packs ought to be available at all healthcare venues, along with posters and emergency help-line numbers.

For community staff visiting people's homes discretion is required if leaving information with the client, especially if the client has limited mobility and finds hiding the information physically impossible. It may be necessary to wait until the client visits the surgery or clinic or until a visit can be arranged when the partner is absent. Especially useful in clinics, surgeries and hospitals are the small adhesive stickers that can be placed on the rear of the toilet door in the Ladies' rest room, one area where men are unable to accompany their partner. Such stickers are available from Women's Aid at a minimal cost and the local refuge number or national help-line number is inserted by staff.

Alternatively, where information sheets, letters, and appointment cards are routinely issued to patients, perhaps the health authority might consider having the local Women's Aid help-line number included for all clients. At ante-natal classes, pregnant women are often given a 'bounty bag', full of leaflets, free samples, etc., in which a small card with the help-line number might be inserted.

Organizations including Women's Aid also provide comprehensive information on their web sites. On-line computers are available for public use in libraries, local colleges, and other public venues, allowing women periodic access to invaluable information. However, if the woman is accessing web pages from a home computer, she ought to be made aware of the safety measures related to Internet use. Most computer software for accessing web pages retains a 'history' record of previous Internet sites visited; the 'history' record can be stored for hours, days, or weeks. In spite of this, it is possible to delete the history immediately after accessing the site, leaving no trace for a suspicious partner to find. Instructions on how to do this can be seen on many web sites dedicated to domestic violence including the Women's Aid Home Page.

Innovative methods of providing information and support to individual clients relevant to their specific health setting are required. Included within an information pack should be a guide to the purchase of safety alarms, either the hand-held alarms that can be purchased in most major shopping centres, or the use of the national care-line scheme. This scheme provides a range of hand-held portable alarms or fixed alarms that can be installed in the house for short periods. Usually there is a monthly charge for the alarms; however, some of these facilities may be available through the local social service department if the woman has limited finances.

Preparing a safety plan

As we have seen previously, for an individual to leave a violent relationship and remain safe she may need to spend a considerable time making plans. Some women are compelled to leave the area where they normally live, often without being able to confide in anyone. Sometimes they are forced to leave behind friends, family, their home and their job. Children too have to leave friends, their school and their family support systems, including a father whom they possibly still love. It is crucial that healthcare staff never under-estimate the lengths to which some men go to retain control of their family and therefore staff have to be in a position to offer the woman advice on how to prepare for the future. An example may be found in Appendix 3.

RISK ASSESSMENT

The concept and practice of risk assessment as it relates to predicting risk behaviours, or personal risk consequences for clients, in areas such as social work, probation services and police work is relatively well established. Undertaking widespread risk assessment has developed more recently in healthcare organizations and usually relates to clinical risk assessment. Assessment of risk behaviours in relation to children and vulnerable persons such as those with mental illness or learning disabilities has evolved within a variety of healthcare settings. However, there is little evidence that risk assessment directly related to domestic abuse has been developed extensively in healthcare.

In domestic violence, there are a number of areas in which undertaking a risk assessment is appropriate. The work on risk assessment in domestic abuse often relates directly to the prediction of the perpetrator's potential for future harming behaviour. This in turn is used to assess the actual and potential risk to the woman and any children within the home and thus determines appropriate intervention strategies.

It is important for healthcare practitioners to be aware of the debate that centres on the effectiveness of risk assessment tools that attempt to predict the future violent and abusive behaviour of individuals. Practitioners need to recognize that risk assessment tools like those used in mental health care settings have limitations when based on statistical prediction.

> The question to be posed in clinical practice is not 'is this person dangerous?' but rather 'might this person in certain circumstances behave in a dangerous way?' (Mullen 1984: 8). Given that these circumstances are likely to be specific to the patient in question, it is important to recognize the value of the idiographic context in making an assessment of risk for a specific patient.
>
> (O'Rourke et al. 2001: 210)

Key point

When seeking to assess the risk of further violence and abuse to the woman and her child or children, never underestimate her ability to determine the level of risk for herself. Whilst she may not articulate this level of risk to others, the woman has undoubtedly developed survival strategies based on her ability to assess and mediate risk. The fact that she has survived so far indicates her ability to deal with the abuse and violence in a way that has as yet kept her alive and not mortally wounded. Therefore, staff should ask the woman for her estimation of future risk based on her past and current experience. Whilst this may underestimate, or even over-estimate, the risk it is nevertheless an important basis from which to begin the assessment. Women have died because others did not hear what they were saying.

A MULTI-AGENCY APPROACH TO RISK MANAGEMENT AND ASSESSMENT

When endeavouring to provide a comprehensive support and protection system for the woman and her children, a collaborative multi-agency approach is the preferred option. This is especially pertinent when undertaking risk assessments. O'Rourke et al. (2001: 5), writing about assessing the risk posed to the general public by clients with mental health illnesses, stated that:

> No agency can operate in isolation when working with risk. The effective management of a person, who presents as a risk to others, cannot just be the responsibility of mental health, social services, or probation or housing. As a public protection issue, it has to be the concern of all agencies, at all levels, and driven as such.

Whilst not implying that an abusive man has a mental health problem, arguably the same principles hold when translated into the work being undertaken by those working collectively to protect and provide a service for abused women. Multi-agency groups have to address the dichotomy that can exist when individual professional identities dictate a code of professional silence known as confidentiality, against the need to share all necessary information required to provide a safe environment for the woman at risk. The forum ought never to lose sight of the fact that every week at least two women in England are murdered by male current or ex-partners.

Risk assessment and child protection

The specific needs of children in abusive homes were addressed in previous chapters where it was seen that a multi-agency, multi-professional child protection service is well established within the UK. However, it is only relatively recently that professionals have recognized that even where no evidence of direct abuse exists, children from violent homes are indirectly suffering abuse and therefore child protection policies may need to be enacted. Indeed, Beattie (1997: 271) believes that: 'Child Protection is an area where professionals have grossly underestimated the risks to children by locating the problem very firmly with women.' It is Beattie's impression that historically women have been persuaded to return to an abusive home or remain within it 'for the sake of the child'. Not surprisingly as more studies are undertaken into domestic violence there is increasing evidence to support the belief that many of the children within these homes also suffer direct abuse from the male partner.

Professionals across disciplines are currently debating how best to deal with children and young people residing in abusive homes even when there is no evidence of direct abuse. On the one hand, those working with women who are being abused advocate an empowering approach that places the women's needs at the centre of intervention strategies. Supportive intervention strategies are structured so that the woman feels empowered to make her own decisions, even if the decision is to stay within the abusive relationship. However, where professionals are required to bring the safety of the children within the home into the equation, there is a likelihood that the solutions required to protect the child will impact on the woman's freedom to choose. On the other hand, accounts of women's experiences indicate that many find the strength to leave because their children are at risk (Beattie 1997: 271), though, equally many do not.

If in the future staff are required to act even without evidence of direct child abuse, there is a serious concern that women may remain silent for fear of involvement of child welfare services, thus exacerbating the silence that already surrounds domestic violence. Nevertheless, those working with women who are being abused need to accept that the safety of the child or children has to be paramount in any intervention strategy. Ahimsa et al. (2002) note that undertaking a risk assessment in these cases can be fraught with difficulty, particularly as it is well recognized that, often, abusive men can be adept at hiding the truth. They note that many of the referrals for risk assessment, particularly when the courts are attempting to make an order about contact, are made to mental health services. However, it is argued that as most men who abuse their partner do not have a psychiatric illness as such, the severity of the risk may go unrecognized.

Women's Aid recommend that risk assessment procedures should be based upon experience in the field and awareness of research into high-risk factors associated with domestic violence. According to Ahimsa (2002): 'Research in fact suggests that *past behaviour alone* may be a better indicator of violence potential than expert opinion based solely upon clinical interview, the results of which many researchers have found to be singularly unimpressive.'

Key points

Undertaking a risk assessment

For an effective risk assessment related to the safety and well-being of the family, to be undertaken for the court it is generally agreed that the following principles should be adhered to.

- The person undertaking the report should have access to ALL relevant documentation including court reports, and medical reports of those concerned.
- Signed consent forms allowing the documents to be released should be obtained prior to the investigation.
- The person undertaking the report must have reasonable access to the accused, the partner and others as appropriate.
- The thoughts and feelings of the individual family members cannot be disregarded when an assessment is undertaken.

Risk assessment and the police services

The MPS in January 2002 piloted a risk assessment form, which after refinement has now been recognized as good practice for police officers. A copy of the form is available on-line at the MPS web site.

Key points

The following are factors that are considered by police when undertaking a risk assessment to determine the potential for a domestic violence perpetrator to re-offend. These factors might be a useful starting-point for healthcare staff, and the multi-agency team attempting to assess existing and future risk to clients presenting with signs of domestic abuse.

The risk categories include whether the perpetrator has a history of:

- previous violence against strangers, acquaintances, family, police officers or animals
- violation of contact and non-contact orders
- recent relationship problems
- recent employment problems
- recent substance abuse/dependence
- recent suicidal or homicidal ideation/intent
- recent psychotic and/or manic symptoms.

continued

Alternatively, whether the perpetrator has a history of past incidents related to:

- domestic abuse events
- sexual assault/sexual jealousy
- use of weapons
- use of threats of death
- escalation in frequency or severity of assaults.

The police also recognize that 'extreme minimization or denial of spousal assault' is a serious cause for concern (MPS 2001).

Risk assessment and staff safety

For staff dealing with clients involved in domestic abuse in the acute phase, for example, in Accident and Emergency departments, the organization ought to be undertaking risk assessments to ensure staff safety. Whilst offenders may not normally offer physical violence to non-intimates it is recognized that their rage can be triggered if an attempt to re-unite with their abused spouse or partner is thwarted. The NHS already acknowledged that healthcare practitioners are increasingly at risk of verbal and physical abuse from clients, with some clients posing a significant safety risk to staff. Therefore, one can justify the implementation of a risk assessment strategy that supports staff working with a client in an abusive relationship where it is anticipated that any healthcare intervention may incur negative responses from the male partner.

Whilst some men who abuse their partners are known to interact with others outside of the home in an aggressive manner, often bullying others to establish or maintain their personal power base, not all are easily recognized as such by outsiders. Therefore, logically healthcare staff involved with the care of abused women and their children are potentially at risk of receiving abuse or violent responses from the clients' partners, and thus the safety of such staff must be paramount.

Risk assessment in refuges

Staff within refuges are well aware of the potential risks of violence both towards residents and to staff and take precautions to maintain a safe environment for everyone involved. The location of refuges is wherever possible kept secret to ensure the women are not harassed or attacked during their stay. Men are not allowed into the refuge and the doors and windows usually have security mechanisms to prevent unlawful entry. Where there is a major safety risk to the woman she may be relocated out of the local area and offered refuge in another town or city. Women living in refuges have to be constantly vigilant when outside the safety of the refuge. They have no way of knowing if they are being followed, or who might pass on their location to the male partner inadvertently or deliberately. Children may have to be kept away from their school for fear that the father is lying in wait at the school gates. If children are re-located, it is essential that staff at the school are made aware of the situation so that information is not inadvertently passed on. Staff within the refuge are well versed in risk assessment and can therefore estimate the potential risk to the individual, her child and other residents.

Risk assessment in probation services

Before a convicted person is released, probation services undertake a risk assessment related to the client's potential to re-offend, including his or her potential for exhibiting violent behaviour in the future if the original offence related to violence. Whilst the probation officer is required to undertake a violence risk assessment on those with a previous history of violence, it is not always known that many of these men may be violent towards their partners. Beattie (1997) expresses concern that there is evidence to show that some intervention strategies dealing with minimizing the man's violence, especially a one-to-one approach, may maintain and even justify the power differentials between men and women. Unless the person working with the perpetrator undertakes appropriate and rigorous training, including an exploration of their own assumptions and values related to their attitudes towards women generally and their roles within relationships specifically, there is a danger that the two may develop a collusive relationship.

Beattie outlines factors that need to be considered when estimating the risk of re-offending, or of perpetrating violent acts even where there is no obvious family history. The probation officer has to consider the perpetrator's past history of violence, especially where it relates to domestic violence. In addition, substance misuse has often been cited as being linked to domestic violence. However, whilst many violent men commit violence under the influence of either drugs or alcohol there is no evidence to show that this is a causal relationship. In fact it is thought that whilst the substances may diminish inhibitions their use is frequently exploited as an excuse by the men to be aggressive and violent (Beattie 1997: 275).

Domestic violence usually escalates in severity over time so that, for example, previous use of a weapon is a strong indicator of the high-risk level in future violent episodes. Studies have also demonstrated that one of the most perilous periods for a woman is the point at which she leaves a violent and abusive relationship. Therefore, any professional undertaking a risk assessment on the man must acknowledge that the loss of his partner and/or the children may trigger an extreme violent reaction against her.

The discourse in the previous chapter showed that most professionals advocate for a feminist-led perpetrator programme, such as that established in Duluth. The Domestic Abuse Intervention Project (DAIP) in Duluth, Minnesota has produced a model of risk assessment that enables staff across the agencies to determine the potential risk of further harm to the abused individual and her child or children.

Staff training and development

Operational progress is inhibited unless staff across agencies and organizations are adequately trained to recognize and assess the risk and to offer alternative interventions. As a minimum requirement the Home Office needs healthcare professionals to be trained to:

- recognize when abuse is occurring and be aware of the wide range of associated issues such as possible reluctance by victims to disclose

- provide sensitive treatment for physical, emotional and psychological injuries including mental health problems brought on as a result of the abuse
- offer support aimed at preventing further injuries
- document the situation, including taking photographs
- assist patients with information about the resources, help and options available to them
- aim to ensure confidentiality and privacy when talking and listening
- safeguard clothing or other evidence that may be required for forensic evidence.

(Home Office 2000b: 2d 6)

Humphreys *et al.* (2001) advise that the effectiveness of domestic violence intervention lies in the development of a comprehensive and widespread training programme. The programme needs to raise awareness amongst all staff and provide adequate training in the skills needed for effective action. The work of Humphreys *et al.* (2000) emphasizes the need for any training to be accompanied by an organizational training strategy that ensures training programmes are cyclical, and require the engagement of staff at all levels. Where possible, training programmes should be run by individuals with the requisite expertise, utilizing outside speakers from, for example, local Women's Aid, refuge workers, DVU police officers or experienced clinicians. Inviting women who have survived abuse to recount their stories and identify needs, can be a compelling learning experience.

The *Good Practice* guidelines authored by Humphreys and colleagues (2001) say what a training programme should offer:

Training to raise awareness, explore values and develop skills. Training needs to include:

1 a strategy for training large numbers of employees in an organization;
2 awareness-raising combined with a range of specialist courses;
3 a rolling programme of domestic violence training;
4 the integration of the training strategy into broader strategic planning for domestic violence intervention;
5 secure financial resources for domestic violence training;
6 attention to training quality.

(Reproduced with permission from Women's Aid Federation of England,
Dr Cathy Humphreys, June 2000a)

In addition, basic awareness training should:

- be extended. After the initial training session other staff may require more in-depth sessions to cover specific issues, including child protection, problems for disabled women, women from ethnic minority groups or identified clinical settings, etc.
- continue over time. All initial training and development programmes in domestic abuse require periodic updating, often on an annual basis if staff are to sustain their original enthusiasm. As new staff are employed they require access to an initial training programme alongside other induction sessions.

In addition, a training programme requires adequate evaluation to ascertain the short- and medium-term effectiveness, followed by a periodic review and further development.

The growth of on-line learning, and the escalating number of sites dedicated to the education of healthcare practitioners, including domestic abuse, if harnessed appropriately can be utilized to extend and enhance the learning opportunities available to staff.

Recognition of the wider implications of domestic abuse, including abuse against all client groups and elder abuse in the home, need to be reflected within training sessions and materials. Training should include the many aspects of care for the woman and her children but it must also include an element of care for the staff member for whom the sessions raise painful or disturbing personal issues. Arguably the training organization has a responsibility to ensure that professional guidance is available for any staff that subsequently feel distressed as a result of the training, or indeed as a result of dealing with clients in abusive relationships.

WORKING TOGETHER TO MAKE A DIFFERENCE

The lack of comprehensive evidence on how the health service could effectively reduce the impact of domestic violence should not be an excuse for lack of action on what we know is a major cause of difficulty for women's health and their quality of life.

(Davidson *et al.* 2000: 3)

Throughout, the need for collaborative working has been emphasized. The problems underpinning domestic abuse cannot be solved unilaterally and the support required by an individual surviving an abusive relationship spans diverse organizations, agencies and voluntary bodies. Although across the country many healthcare practitioners and small groups are making a difference, historically healthcare professionals have not been leaders in the field of inter-agency innovative practice.

With the raising of the international profile of domestic violence and abuse, it is time for health services across Britain to recognize that the consequences of inaction in the past have culminated in a major public health deficit for the women, children and men continually forced to share their living spaces with violent and abusive intimates. What is urgently required is a systematic review of each healthcare setting to determine existing deficits. Once this is completed the organization should be required to have in place planned and structured resolutions that offer individuals protection and the support they need to survive and eventually establish a life outside of the relationship. Staff ought to feel confident to work with clients within an abusive relationship, and have the knowledge of what to do, the skills to put it into practice and the supplementary resources to enact the plan of action.

Equally it is important for staff to be confident that the resources are in place for their personal support and guidance, in order that the job can be accomplished without emotional and psychological harm to them. Good practice demands that all healthcare organizations provide policies and services to support staff who find themselves living in an abusive relationship.

Appendices

The details of the following resources were correct at the time of publication in February 2004.

Photocopiable
Resource

Indicates that this resource page may be photocopied for use by practitioners.

Key resources

Photocopiable
Resource

National helpline numbers for clients include:

Women's Aid National Domestic Violence Helpline
Tel: 0808 2000 247 (24-hr)

Scotland Domestic Abuse National Helpline
Tel: 0800 027 1234 (24-hr)

Northern Ireland Women's Aid Helpline
Tel: 028 90 331818 (24-hr)

Republic of Ireland Women's Aid Helpline
Tel: 1800 341900 (10 a.m.–10 p.m.)

Welsh Women's Aid Helpline
Tel: 02920 390874

Victim Supportline National Helpline
Tel: 0845 3030900
9 a.m.–9 p.m. weekdays, 9 a.m.–7 p.m. weekends, 9 a.m.–5 p.m. bank holidays

Refuge National Domestic Violence Helpline
Tel: 0870 599 5443 (24-hr)

The Samaritans
Tel: 08457 909090 (24-hr)

ChildLine
Tel: 0800 1111 (24-hr line for children to use)

London Lesbian and Gay Switchboard National Helpline
Tel: 020 7837 7324

© Routledge 2004

Photocopiable
Resource

Women's Aid

Women's Aid National Office
PO Box 391
Bristol BS99 7WS
Tel: 0117 944 4411 (office)

**Women's Aid Refuge
Republic of Ireland**
Rathmines
Dublin 6
Tel: 00 353 1 496 1002

Scottish Women's Aid
Norton Park
57 Albion Road
Edinburgh EH7 5QY
Tel: 01 31 475 2372

London Women's Aid
PO Box 14041
London E1 6NY
Tel: 020 7392 2092 (24-hr helpline)

Northern Ireland Women's Aid Federation
129 University Street
Belfast BT7 1HP
Tel: 02890 249 041

Welsh Women's Aid (Aberystwyth)
4 Pound Place
Aberystwyth SY23 1LX
Tel: 02920 390874

Victim Support

**Victim Support England & Wales
(national office)**
Cranmer House
39 Brixton Road
London SW9 6DZ
Tel: 020 7735 9166

Victim Support Scotland
15–23 Hardwell Close
Edinburgh EH8 9RX
Tel: 0131 668 4486
info@victimsupportsco.demon.co.uk

Refuge
2–8 Maltravers Street
London WC2 3EE
Tel: 0207 395 7700

Victim Support Northern Ireland
Annsgate House
70–4 Ann Street
Belfast BT1 4EH
Tel: 01232 244039

Victim Support (Republic of Ireland)
Haliday House
Dublin 7
Eire
Tel: 00 353 1 8780870

Southall Black Sisters
52 Norwood Road
Southall
Middlesex UB2 4DW
Tel: 0208 571 9595 (office closed Weds)

Photocopiable
Resource

Refugee Women's Resource Project
c/o Asylum Aid
28 Commercial Street
London E1 6LS
Tel: 020 7377 51 2 3
rwrp@asylumaid.org.uk
Provides free legal representation and
advice to asylum seekers and refugees.
It aims to enable women fleeing serious
human rights violations to gain
protection in the UK

Immigration Advisory Service
Tel: 020 7378 91 91 .
24-hr helpline for advice about immigration,
asylum rules and the law

Survivors
For men who have been raped
PO Box 2470
London W2 1NW
Helpline 02 07-357 6677
W: www.survivorsuk.co.uk
E: Info@survivorsuk.org.uk

Jewish Women's Aid
Tel: 020 84458060
Email: jwa@dircon.co.uk
www.jwauk.cjb.net

SOLA
**(Survivors of Lesbian Partnership
Abuse)**
Helpline: 020 7328 7389
E-mail : solalondon@hotmail.com
London-based group SOLA offer
support to women who have been
abused by a female (ex-)partner

Broken Rainbow Hotline
Tel: 07 812 644 914
A reporting and referral service for lesbians,
gay men, bisexuals and transgender people
experiencing domestic violence

Shelterline
Tel: 0808 800 4444
24-hr national housing advice line
www.shelternet.org.uk

For children

National Child Protection Helpline
Tel: 0800 800500 (24-hr)

Careline Confidential
Telephone counselling for children, young
people and adults:
020 8514 1177

Photocopiable
Resource

Rape and Sexual Assault contacts

Rape Crisis Federation Wales and England
Unit 7 Provident Works
Newdigate Street
Nottingham NG7 4FD
Tel: 0115 900 3560
Fax: 0115 900 3562
Minicom: 0115 900 3563
Email: info@rapecrisis.co.uk

Central Scotland Rape Crisis & Sexual Abuse Centre
PO Box 48
Stirling, FK8 1YG
PO Box 38
Falkirk, FK1 1AA
Helpline: 01786 471771

Rape Crisis Federation Ireland
7 Francis Street
Galway
Eire
Tel: 091 563676
Email: ncci@tinet.ie

Domestic Violence Programmes

Domestic Abuse Intervention Project (DAIP)
202 East Superior Street
Duluth
Minnesota 55802
www.duluth-model.org

Shelter
(homeless needs)
National help-line: 0800 446 441

Domestic Violence Intervention Programme (DVIP)
PO Box 2838
London W6 9ZE
Email: info@dvip.org
Provides a range of diverse services –
perpetrator programmes for violent men and
support services for women and children.

Good practice indicators from WAFE

The good practice indicators have been written to provide standards through which organizations can check their domestic violence service developments. The indicators are provisional with room for more specific refinements in the future. Reproduced with permission from Women's Aid Federation of England, Dr Cathy Humphreys, 'Child Protection and Woman Protection: Links and Schisms. An Overview of the Research', June 2000, WAFE web page.

These indicators were developed alongside the mapping of service provision in the UK and include:

Framework of indicators

A definition of domestic violence, which sets the parameters for policy and practice development in the organization and in the multi-agency context.

1 **Definitions need to:**

   a) acknowledge diversity, acknowledge the gendered nature of domestic violence and include different types of abuse;
   b) provide recognition of domestic violence as an abuse of power and control of one person by another.

2 **Monitoring and screening for domestic violence through:**

   a) systematic screening, using a protocol of questions which emphasize particular behaviours, rather than initially asking directly about domestic violence;
   b) mechanisms for recording domestic violence;
   c) guidance and supervision for front-line practitioners;
   d) training associated with the introduction of screening and monitoring;
   e) feedback mechanisms for using the monitoring data.

3 **Policies and guidelines which provide a framework for the work to be undertaken**

Policies need to:

   a) emphasize safety and clarify issues of confidentiality;
   b) give attention to diversity and equalities issues;

c) involve survivors of domestic violence and their representatives in refuge and advocacy services;
d) develop policies particular to the organization, in conjunction with a wider multi-agency strategy;
e) children and families, vulnerable adults, community care recipients and perpetrators; practice guidelines for front-line workers; safety policies for workers; and policies specific to the service provided by each department and organization;
f) embed policies within the organization, through training, guidance, the development of appropriate procedures and service provision;
g) detailed guidelines which explicate the issues for practice.

4   Safety measures and planning to include:

a) safety planning with individuals who may face violence and abuse;
b) ensuring the safety of women and children through a range of measures at organizational level aimed at stopping violence or minimizing risk;
c) supporting and ensuring the safety of mothers as a means of protecting and enhancing the welfare of children;
d) organizational measures to ensure workers' safety.

5   Training to raise awareness, explore values and develop skills

Training needs to include:

a) a strategy for training large numbers of employees in an organization;
b) awareness-raising combined with a range of specialist courses;
c) a rolling programme of domestic violence training;
d) the integration of the training strategy into broader strategic planning for domestic violence intervention;
e) secure financial resources for domestic violence training;
f) attention to training quality.

6   Evaluation

The framework of indicators listed above provides parameters for evaluation, with different considerations applying to evaluating work with survivors, on the one hand, and work with perpetrators, on the other. Sub-indicators of good practice in respect of evaluation in the field of domestic violence have been identified as the following:

a) independent evaluation conducted by researchers with expertise in the domestic violence area;
b) building-in the voice of survivors in respect of work with women and/or children;
c) follow-up to ensure that women and children remain safe;
d) feedback loop to examine what works and also to identify areas of practice which need to change.

7   Multi-agency strategy to co-ordinate the development of policy and practice across organizations within an area. The strategy should include:

a) attention to consistency of services and policies across and within agencies;
b) attention to issues of confidentiality and permission;
c) full and active involvement of women's refuge, outreach and support services;
d) attention to equalities issues and effective mechanisms for consultation with service users;
e) clarity about decisions, actions and accountability;
f) monitoring of the effectiveness and evaluation of interagency co-ordination;
g) measurable improvements in resourcing.

8 Guidelines for working with domestic violence survivors (usually women and children). All practice interventions need to include a practical focus on the needs of women and children experiencing domestic violence. While all the above dimensions of good practice will apply, other sub-indicators for practice interventions will include the underpinning of work by the assumption that supporting women is often an effective means of supporting and protecting children, while acknowledging that children's and women's needs and experiences are different and require separate, but linked, provision. The sub-indicators include:

a) attention to the voices and expressed needs of women using the service, so that provision is sensitively attuned to these needs;
b) attention to children's needs in terms of preventative work on abuse with children, as well as child protection issues;
c) the empowerment of abused women and children so that they are enabled to build effective responses to abuse and positive future lives;
d) attempts to mainstream the service, so that concrete and empowering work with abused women and children spreads across all sectors;
e) monitoring and evaluation to ensure effective provision;
f) cost-effectiveness in order to best use available resources.

9 General principles underlying all provision and service development with abused women and children include:

a) the first and main priority to be improvements in safety;
b) the adoption of a believing, sensitive approach;
c) the provision and delivery of a range of services, including safe house accommodation, advocacy, outreach, and housing services;
d) the development of specific and diverse services in relation to minority ethnic and other communities.

Reproduced with kind permission of WAFE (2001)

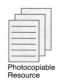

Photocopiable
Resource

Appendix 3

Devising a safety plan

Devise a safety plan

Planning a safe exit from the relationship enables a woman to take some control over a potentially dangerous situation in addition to giving her a sense of a better future. Women should know that it is often possible to make contact with the local domestic violence unit (DVU) or the domestic violence officer (DVO) at the local police station at any point during the relationship. Thus the police are aware of the inherent dangers to the woman, and they have a record of previous abuse incidents. The woman needs to be reassured that no action will be taken without her express wish to proceed unless and until an incident occurs in which she or one of her children is injured.

Women in abusive relationships should be advised to:

- Find a safe place, possibly with a close friend or relative where she can store clothes and valuables for a period. If possible, the items should be kept away from the shared home.
- Gradually put a few clothes for herself and any children in a bag in the place of safety, any valuables that will not be missed, and even a few of the children's small toys.
- Consider the possibility of purchasing a mobile phone if she does not already have one.
- Either store original copies of important documents in a place with easy access in the home, or if it is safe to do so, put them in the place of safety. Alternatively if the original documents would be easily missed by the partner, photocopies should be made and hidden. Documents might include:

  - passport
  - birth certificates
  - driving licence
  - marriage certificate
  - bank details
  - children's medical records, immunizations, etc.
  - national insurance cards
  - address book
  - letters, etc., that might identify the place of safety

- If the woman is in possession of a court order banning the man from entering the house, approaching or molesting her, then she should keep it readily available or leave it with a close friend while keeping a copy in her own possession.

Photocopiable
Resource

- Make copies of keys including house and car keys and keep them in a place that is easy to access if there is an urgent need to leave the house. An abusive man will often confiscate keys as a means of control, when to do so means the woman cannot return to the house even in his absence.
- Compile and keep a list of helping agencies including the local women's refuge, the emergency help-line numbers.
- Plan an escape route if possible, by making advance contingency plans as to where she could stay, whom with, how she would get there, with whom it would be safe to share the information.
- Remedications for self or children, it may be possible to obtain a prescription from the GP for any regular medication that can be used during an emergency.

Safety during a violent episode

There are a number of things a woman might consider doing to protect herself during a violent episode including:

- discussing in advance with the children (depending of course on their age) what steps they might take in such an event. This may include ensuring they leave the house immediately if the mother tells them to do so, and if possible alerting a neighbour in advance.
- Having a 'hot-key' for the emergency services on the telephone or mobile and carrying the mobile whenever it is possible.
- Avoiding being trapped in a room with no exit or a room that can be locked from either side, such as a bedroom.
- It may be advisable for her to test out the escape plan prior to actually needing to use it.

Safety after the 'event'

We have already seen that the most dangerous time for a woman in an abusive relationship is often at the point of her leaving, or just after she has left. Therefore, if it is feasible, planning an escape would be the most effective way of exiting the relationship without harm.

Even though the woman has somewhere to stay it may be crucial that she reside in a refuge for a short period, as the partner is less likely to find her or be able to contact her.

Advice from the Royal College of General Practitioners

No patient should ever be pressurized into following any particular course of action. Only the patient can decide what is right for her in her particular situation. Her individual autonomy, self-esteem and self-determination should be encouraged and respected. Even if the patient decides to return to the violent situation, she is not likely to forget the information and care given and, in time, this may help her to break out of the cycle of abuse. Beware of the danger that the needs of some ethnic minority patients may be ignored under the guise of 'respect' for different cultures.

Photocopiable
Resource

1   If she does not wish to return to the abuser, advise her on the services available from local agencies and offer help with contacting them.

2   If she chooses to return to the abuser:

   (a) Give her the telephone number of the local women's refuge or the local Women's Aid.

   (b) Advise her to keep some money and important financial and legal documents hidden in a safe place, in case of emergency.

   (c) Help her to plan an escape route in case of emergency.

3   If children are likely to be at risk, seriously consider referral to social services, if possible with the patient's consent.

Reprinted with permission from the Royal College of General Practitioners, Dr Iona Heath, MRCP, FRCGP, 'Domestic Violence: the General Practitioner's Role'

Social Service Inspection Standards

1: Children Act principles

The SSD actively promotes the principles of the Children Act through its policy, procedures and practice, and there are management arrangements in place to monitor their effectiveness.

2: Equal opportunities

Family support services positively attempt to meet the needs and preferences of children and families in respect of race, religion, language, culture, gender and disability, supported by policies and procedures. SSD staff advocate that all other professional people involved with the families take these issues into account.

3: Policy

The Local Authority has a clearly written, comprehensive policy for planning and provision of family support services.

4: Onter-agency collaboration in planning and service delivery

The Local Authority ensures collaboration with other agencies and authorities in its area in the planning, development, resourcing, delivery, evaluation and review of family support services.

5: Management

The SSD's family support services are delivered through integrated management structures and procedures which ensure that the service response to the multiple needs of each child and family is co-ordinated.

6: Access to service

The Local Authority SSD provides information to the public and others about the availability of family support services, eligibility criteria and arrangements for access to them.

7: Receiving referrals and determining the level of response

The SSD has clear and sensitive arrangements for receiving and acting on a referral regarding an individual child's family which, on the basis of an initial identification of need, determines risk, eligibility, priority and speed of response.

8: Assessment

The SSD undertakes a range of initial and further assessments to determine the extent and type of services which are required to meet the needs of children and their families in individual cases.

9: Decision-making

Decisions about cases reflect SSD policy, procedures and practice guidance in respect of risk eligibility and provision of services and are based on accurate, early assessment of need, and professional judgements.

10: Planning

Where a service is to be provided a recorded plan is constructed with the involvement of the family and child, other carers and relevant agencies. The initial plan is revised in the light of changing circumstances.

11: Service provision

Services provided to individual families derive from their plan and are co-ordinated with existing and potential providers. The services are designed to be flexible and to use resources creatively in ways which best meet the needs and preferences of the children and families.

12: Staff competence and deployment

The SSD has in place a human resource strategy which ensures that its workforce is appropriately trained, deployed and supported, and has clear expectations of other providers to work to the same standards.

'SSI Inspection of Assessment, Planning and Decision-Making in Family Support Services'. Classification: Children and young people. Reproduced with permission from the Department of Health.
First use: 1998

The Domestic Abuse Intervention Project (DAIP) in Duluth, Minnesota: a guide to practice

Risk assessment questions

The Duluth Domestic Abuse Intervention Project (DAIP) has developed a risk assessment questionnaire based on current research and years of interviews with victims of domestic violence, police and probation officers, mental health workers, public health nurses, and victim advocates. The following is offered as a guide for development locally and as one might expect, the questions are similar to findings in a range of UK literature on the subject.

The role of the healthcare provider in this process needs to be determined at a local level. Whilst it is acknowledged that healthcare professionals must be pro-active in the assessment, planning and intervention of domestic abuse, a successful approach is one that is co-ordinated across disciplines. Therefore, the following is offered as a basis from which local policies and protocols might be developed rather than as a tool to be used indiscriminately by individual practitioners.

The Duluth Domestic Abuse Intervention Project (DAIP) risk assessment

1   Has the abuser become increasingly more violent, brutal, and/or dangerous? Can you describe the incident? What do you think that change in behaviour means?
2   Has the abuser ever injured you so badly you needed medical attention? Can you describe the injuries? Have they become increasingly more severe? Are you concerned about what will happen next?
3   Has the abuser ever choked you? Can you describe the incident? Did you lose consciousness?
4   Has the abuser ever injured or killed a pet? Can you describe the incident? Do you think he did it to threaten you?
5   Has the abuser ever threatened to kill you? Can you describe the incident? Do you believe he is willing and capable of carrying out that threat?
6   Has the abuser been sexually abusive to you?
7   Has the abuser used or threatened to use a weapon against you? Can you describe the incident/s? Do you think he may use a weapon against you?
8   Has the abuser seemed preoccupied or obsessed with you (e.g., following you, monitoring your whereabouts, stalking you, very jealous)? Can you describe the behaviour?

9   Has the abuser increased the frequency of assaults on [his] victim? Can you describe the pattern?

10 Has the abuser ever threatened or attempted to commit suicide? Can you describe the incident? How did that [a]ffect you?

11 Have you separated or tried to separate from the abuser in the past twelve months? Can you describe how that went?

12 Have you sought outside help (e.g., a protection order, police, shelter, counselling) during the past twelve months? Can you tell me how he responded to that?

13 Do you think you have been isolated from sources of help (car, phone, family, friends, etc.)? Can you give me an idea of how he responds to your efforts to reach out for help?

14 Has the abuser experienced any unusual high stress in the past twelve months (e.g., loss of job, death, financial crisis)? Do you think that has made him any more dangerous to you?

15 Does the abuser drink excessively/have an alcohol problem? What is the relationship of his drinking to his violence?

16 Has the abuser ever been treated for alcohol/drug abuse? How do you think that [a]ffects his use of violence?

17 Does the abuser own, carry, or have ready access to a gun? Specify.

18 Do you believe the abuser could seriously injure or kill you?

19 Have you felt a need to be protective of the abuser (e.g., tried to change or withdraw [a] statement to the police, reduce bail or charges)?

20 To the best of your knowledge, was the abuser abused as a child by a family member? Can you tell me more information about that?

21 To the best of your knowledge, did the abuser witness the physical abuse of his mother? Do you think that's connected to his use of violence now?

22 Does the abuser show remorse or sadness about the incident?

23 Does the abuser have a history of violence to others (i.e., persons outside the family)? Can you describe this?

Reproduced with permission from the Duluth Domestic Abuse Intervention Project (DAIP), Minnesota, USA

'Domestic Violence: the General Practitioner's Role': an extract

This extract is reproduced with the permission of the Royal College of General Practitioners from the work of Dr Iona Heath, MRCP, FRCGP

Consider the possibility of domestic violence if:

The possibility of domestic violence should be considered in any of the following situations:

1 Patient admits to past or present abuse.
2 Patient presents with unexplained bruises, whiplash injuries consistent with shaking, areas of erythema consistent with slap injuries, lacerations, burns or multiple injuries in various stages of healing.
3 Patient presents with injuries to areas hidden by clothing (Mehta and Dandrea 1988). Note that it can be very easy not to examine, for example, first generation Asian women properly because of their apparent shyness and because of the sometimes unfamiliar nature of their clothing.
4 Patient presents with injuries to face, chest, breast and abdomen (Stark *et al.* 1979).
5 Patient presents evidence of sexual abuse.
6 Extent or type of injury is inconsistent with explanation by patient.
7 Substantial delay exists between time of injury and presentation for treatment.
8 Patient describes the alleged 'accident' in hesitant, embarrassed or evasive manner.
9 Review of medical record reveals that patient has presented with repeated 'accidental' injuries.
10 Patient presents repeatedly with physical symptoms for which no explanation can be found (Jaffe *et al.* 1976). This presentation may be particularly common among women whose first language is not English, and who therefore may find it difficult to express their feelings and suffering (Fenton and Sadiq 1993).
11 Partner accompanies patient, insists on staying close to patient and answers all questions.
12 Patient is pregnant (Mezey and Bewley 1997). Domestic violence often begins with the first pregnancy. Injuries are most commonly to the breasts or abdomen (Lent 1991).
13 Patient has history of miscarriage. Women experiencing domestic violence are 15 times more likely to have suffered a miscarriage (Stark and Flitcraft 1996).
14 History of psychiatric illness, alcohol or drug dependence in patient or partner (Jaffe *et al.* 1986; Andrews and Brown 1988).

15   History of attempted suicide (Gayford 1975; Stark *et al.* 1979). In the USA, domestic violence accounts for one in four suicide attempts by women.

16   History of depression, anxiety, failure to cope, social withdrawal, with underlying sense of helplessness.

17   History of behaviour problems or unexplained injuries or abuse affecting children (Mehta and Dandrea 1988; Abrahams 1994).

Advice from the Royal College of General Practitioners

No patient should ever be pressurized into following any particular course of action. Only the patient can decide what is right for her in her particular situation. Her individual autonomy, self-esteem and self-determination should be encouraged and respected. Even if the patient decides to return to the violent situation, she is not likely to forget the information and care given and, in time, this may help her to break out of the cycle of abuse. Beware of the danger of the needs of some ethnic minority patients being ignored under the guise of 'respect' for different cultures.

- If she does not wish to return to the abuser, advise her on the services available from local agencies and offer help with contacting them.

- If she chooses to return to the abuser:

- (a) Give her the telephone number of the local women's refuge or the local Women's Aid.

- (b) Advise her to keep some money and important financial and legal documents hidden in a safe place, in case of emergency.

- (c) Help her to plan an escape route in case of emergency.

- If children are likely to be at risk, seriously consider referral to social services, if possible with the patient's consent.

Reprinted with permission from the RCGP: Dr Iona Heath, MRCP, FRCGP, 'Domestic Violence: the General Practitioner's Role'

References

Abrahams, C. *The Hidden Victims: Children and Domestic Violence.* London: NCH Action for Children, 1994.

Andrews, B. and Brown, G.W. 'Marital violence in the community'. *British Journal of Psychiatry 153,* 305–12, 1988.

Fenton, S. and Sadiq, A. (eds) *The Sorrow in My Heart: sixteen Asian women speak about depression.* London: Commission for Racial Equality, 1993.

Gayford, J.J. 'Wife battering: a preliminary survey of 100 cases'. *British Medical Journal 1,* 194–7, 1975.

Jaffe, P., Wolfe, D.A., Wilson, S. *et al.* 'Emotional and physical health problems of battered women'. *Canadian Journal of Psychiatry 31,* 625–9, 1986.

Lent, B. (ed) *Reports on Wife Assault.* Ontario: Ontario Medical Association Committee on Wife Assault, 1991.

Mehta, P. and Dandrea, L. 'The battered woman'. *American Family Physician 37,* 193–9, 1988.

Mezey, G. and Bewley, G. C., 'Domestic Violence and Pregnancy: Risk Is Greatest after Delivery' [Editorial], *British Medical Journal*, *314(7090)*, p. 1295, 3 May 1997.

Stark, E. and Flitcraft, A., *Women at Risk: Domestic Violence and Women's Health*. Sage, London 1996.

Stark, E., Flitcraft, A. and Frazier, W., 'Medicine and Patriarchal Violence: the Social Construction of a "Private Event"', *Int. Journal of Health Services*, *9(3)*, pp. 461–93, 1979.

'Domestic Violence: the General Practitioner's Role': an extract on photographic evidence

This extract is reproduced with the permission of the Royal College of General Practitioners from the work of Dr Iona Heath, MRCP, FRCGP, 'Domestic Violence: The General Practitioner's Role'

Photographs

Photographs can convey the severity of injuries much more effectively than verbal description and, whenever possible, photographs should be taken of all patients with visible injuries. This will not be possible for many general practitioners and, if this is the case, advise the patient to have photographs taken elsewhere.

1 Explain to the patient that photographs will be very useful as evidence if she decides to prosecute the abuser now or in the future.
2 Explain to the patient that photographs will become part of the patient's medical record and, as such, can only be released with the patient's permission.
3 Obtain written consent from the patient to take photographs. (Written informed consent should include the statement, 'These photographs will only be released if and when the undersigned gives written permission to release the medical records'.)
4 Use a good Polaroid camera with colour film flash bulbs.
5 Photograph in brightest light possible.
6 Attempt to take close-up of injury but try to include an identifiable feature of the patient. If this is not possible, a long shot should be followed by a close-up.
7 The photographer should sign and date the back of each photograph.
8 Place photographs in a sealed envelope and attach securely to the patient's record. Mark the envelope with the date and the notation 'Photographs of patient's injuries'.
9 Bruising is often more obvious two or three days after the injury. If this is likely to be the case, the patient should be advised to return at a later date, or to have more photographs taken elsewhere (for example, at the police station).

Key web resources

Photocopiable Resource

The following Web Page references are accurate at the time of publication.

American Medical Association (AMA)	515 N. State Street Chicago, IL 60610 http://www.ama-assn.org/
Cabinet Office (1999) *Living without fear*	http://www.cabinet-office.gov.uk/ womensunit/1999/fear/index/htm
Center for Research on Women with Disabilities	http://www.bcm.tmc.edu/crowd/index.htm
Centre for Prevention of Sexual and Domestic Violence	http://www.cpsdv.org
Coventry Domestic Violence Group provide excellent information on the needs of children and young people	http://www.coventry.gov.uk/social/child/ dome/index.html
Crown Prosecution Services	http://www.cps.gov.uk/
Department of Health	http://www.doh.gov.uk/
Domestic Abuse Intervention Project (DAIP)	http://www.duluth-model.org
Domestic Violence Intervention Project (DVIP)	http://www.dvip.org
Domestic Violence resources (OMNI)	http://omni.ac.uk/subject-listing/HQ809.html
European Parliament, Women's Lobby	http://nt.oneworld.nl/ewlobby/en/themes/ violence/public_bon.html Contact: centre-violence@womenlobby.org
Family Law information	http://www.legalday.co.uk/indx/family.shtml
Family Violence Prevention Fund's National Health Resource Center on Domestic Violence (USA)	http//www.fvpf.org
Home Office	http://www.homeoffice.gov.uk/
Home Office (2000)	http://www.homeoffice.gov.uk/ domesticviolence/brief.htm
Jewish Women Organisation	http://www.jewishwomen.org/Relationship

Photocopiable
Resource

Joseph Rowntree Foundation	http://www.jrf.org.uk/home.asp
Lord Chancellors Department: Family & Individual matters	http://www.lcd.gov.uk/family/famfr.htm
Metropolitan Police Service	http://www.met.police.uk/
Male abuse information site	http://www.wadv.org/maleabuse.htm
Newham Domestic Violence Forum Directory	http://www.newhamdvf.org.uk/Home.html
NCH a wide variety of resources about children and young people	http://www.nch.org.uk/
Northern Ireland Womens Aid Federation	http://www.niwaf.org/index.htm
Rape Crisis Federation Wales & England	http://www.rapecrisis.co.uk/
Supporting people – housing	http://www.spkweb.org.uk/
Royal College of General Practitioners (including specific advice when children are in the home)	http://www.rcgp.org.uk/index.asp http://www.rcgp.org.uk/rcgp/corporate/ position/dom_viol_families/coexist.asp
Royal College of Nursing	http://www.rcn.org.uk/
Royal College of Midwives	http://www.rcm.org.uk/
School Nurse and Health Visitor Innovation Projects	http://www.innovate.hda.online.org.uk
Survivors – a male rape help line	http://www.survivorsuk.co.uk/ info@survivorsuk.org.uk
Survive-UK for survivors of rape and serious sexial assault	http://survive.org.uk/indexx.html
UK Disability Forum – information for disabled women in abusive relationships	http://www.edfwomen.org.uk/abuse.htm
Victim Support England & Wales	http://www.victimsupport.org.uk
Victim Support Northern Ireland	EMAIL: info@victimsupport.ie Web Site: http://www.victimsupport.ie/
Women's Aid Federation of England	http://www.womensaid.org.uk/
Women and Equality Unit	http://www.womens-unit.gov.uk/ domestic_violence/index.htm
World Health Organisation (Europe)	http://www.who.dk
Women and Equality Unit	www.womenandequalityunit.gov.uk
World Health Organisation Women's pages	http://www.oms.ch/frh-whd/

References

Abbasi, K., 'Obstetricians Must Ask about Domestic Violence', *BMJ*, 316(7), 3 January 1998.

Abbott, P. and Williamson, E., 'Women, Health and Domestic Violence', *Journal of Gender Studies*, 8(1), pp. 83–102, 1999.

Ahimsa (2002) *Risk Assessments Conducted by Ahimsa and Related to Child Welfare Proceedings*. Available online: http://www.ahimsa.org.uk/docs/riskprfr.htm

American Federation of State, County and Municipal Employees (AFSCME), 2000: http://www.afscme.org/health/viol06.htm

American Medical Association (AMA), *Diagnostic and Treatment Guidelines on Domestic Violence*. AMA, Chicago, 1992.

American Medical Association, *Strategies for the Prevention and Management of Sexual Assault*. American Medical Association 515 N. State Street Chicago, IL 60610. Chicago 1995a. http://www.ama-assn.org/

American Medical Association, *Diagnostic and Treatment Guidelines on Mental Health Effects of Family Violence*. 515 N. State Street Chicago, IL 60610. Chicago 1995b. http://www.ama-assn.org/

American Psychiatric Association, *Diagnostic and Statistical Manual of Mental Disorders*, 4th edn (DSM IV). APA, Washington DC 1994.

Antonelli, J. S. and Pearl, A., San Francisco Jewish Community Publications Inc., *Jewish Bulletin of Northern California*. 12 January 1996. http://www.jewishsf.com/bk960112/pagehome.htm

Association for Genitourinary Medicine (AGUM), *UK National Guidelines on Sexually Transmitted Infections and Closely Related Conditions Clinical Effectiveness Group Association for Genitourinary Medicine (AGUM)*. Medical Society for the Study of Venereal Diseases (MSSVD).

Atkins, S. and Hoggett, B., *Women and the Law*. Blackwell, London, 1984.

Augenbraun, M., Wilson, T. E. and Allister, L., 'Domestic Violence reported by Women attending a Sexually Transmitted Disease Clinic', *American Sexually Transmitted Diseases Association*, 28(3), pp. 143–7, March 2001.

Awake: Watch Tower Bible and Tract Society of Pennsylvania, 2001. Watchtower http://www.watchtower.org/

Barnet, O. W., Miller-Perrin, C. L. and Perrin, R. D., *Family Violence across the Lifespan: an Introduction*. Sage, London 1997.

Bartal, B. F., *The British Criminology Conferences: Selected Proceedings. Volume 1: Emerging Themes in Criminology*. In Vagg, J. and Newburn, T. (eds). Papers from the British Criminology Conference, Loughborough University, 18–21 July 1995. This volume published September 1998.

BBC on-line, *UK Homeless Women blame Domestic Violence*, Sunday, 30 May 1999.

Beattie, K., 'Risk Domestic Violence and Probation Practice'. In Kemshall, H., Pritchard, J. (eds), *Good Practice in Risk Assessment and Risk Management 2*, Chapter 17. Jessica Kingsley Publications, London 1997.

Berios, D. C. and Grady, D., 'Domestic Violence: Risk Factors and Outcome', *The Western Journal of Medicine*, 155(2), August 1991.

Berry, D. B., *The Domestic Violence Sourcebook*, 3rd edn. Lowell House, Los Angeles 2000.

Bloomington, M. N., *Institute for Clinical Systems Improvement* (ICSI), Nov. 2001, p. 39 available at http://www.health.org/catalog/catalog.htm

Bradley, F., Smith, M., Long J. and O'Dowd, T., 'Reported Frequency of Domestic Violence: Cross Sectional Survey of Women attending General Practice', *British Medical Journal*, 324(7332), pp. 271–3, 2 February 2002.

Brandon, M. and Lewis, A., 'Significant Harm and Children's Experiences of Domestic Violence', *Child and Family Social Work, 1*, pp. 33–42, 1996.

British Association of Accident and Emergency Medicine (BAAEM), 1990 Central Consultants and Specialists Committee (CCSC), *Police Requests for Information from Medical Practitioners in Hospital Accident and Emergency Departments Guidance for Consultants, or Other Doctors In Charge of Accident and Emergency Departments*. London, BAAEM at the Royal College of Surgeons of England 1990: http://www.baem.org.uk/ccsc.htm

British Association of Accident and Emergency Medicine, *DOMESTIC VIOLENCE: Recognition and Management in Accident and Emergency*. London, BAAEM at the Royal College of Surgeons of England 1993: http://www.baem.org.uk/ccsc.htm

British Medical Association (BMA), *Domestic Violence: a Health Care Issue?* BMA, London 1999.

Brown, K., Johnson, F., Tuohy, M., Watson, J. and Watts, S., *Domestic Violence: a Training Pack for Health Professionals*. Camden Multi-agency Domestic Violence Forum, London 1999.

Budd, T. and Mattinson J., *The Extent and Nature of Stalking: Findings from the 1998 British Crime Survey*. Home Office RDSD Research Findings No. 129. London 2000.

Burge, S., 'Violence against Women as a Health Care Issue', *Family Medicine, 21*, pp. 368–73, 1989.

Burke, T. W., 'Male-to-Male Gay Domestic Violence: the Dark Closet', Chapter 7 in Jackson, A. J. and Oates, G. C., *Violence in Intimate Relationships: Examining Sociological and Psychological Issues*. Butterworth-Heinemann, Oxford and Boston 1998.

Burton, S., Regan, L. and Kelly, L., *Supporting Women and Challenging Men: Lessons from the Domestic Violence Intervention Project*. Policy Press, London 1998.

Butler, M. J., 'Domestic Violence: a Nursing Imperative', *Journal of Holistic Nursing, 13(1)*, pp. 54–69, 1995.

Camden Domestic Violence Health Project, *The Response of Health Professionals to Domestic Violence*. Camden Council Equalities Unit, London 1998.

Campbell, J. C., 'Nursing Assessments for Risk of Homicide with Battered Women', *Advances in Nursing Science, 8(4)*, pp. 36–51, 1986.

Carlson, B. E., 'Adolescent Observers of Marital Violence', *Journal of Family Violence, 7*, pp. 249–59, 1990.

Centre for Prevention of Sexual and Domestic Violence, 'What Every Congregation needs to know about Domestic Violence', Centre for Prevention of Sexual and Domestic Violence (CPSDV), Seattle October 1994. www.cpsdv.org

Chavez, L. J., *Domestic Violence, a Puzzling Issue for Employers*. Hostage Negotiator, Sacramento Police Department, 1996: http://www.workplace-violence.com/

Clarkson, C., Cretney, A., Davis, G. and Shepherd, J. P., 'Assault: the Relationship between Seriousness, Criminalisation and Punishment', *Criminal Law Review*, pp. 4–20, 4 January 1994.

Community Practitioners and Health Visitors Association (CPHVA), *Keeping the Record Straight*. CPHVA, London 1998.

Corrigan, S., *'Caught in the Middle'. Exploring Children and Young People's Experience of Domestic Violence*. Northern Ireland Women's Aid Federation, Belfast 1998.

Covington, D. L., Dalton, V. K., Diehl, S. J., Wright, B. D. and Piner, M. H., 'Improving Detection of Violence amongst Pregnant Adolescents . . . Systematic Violence Assessment', *Journal of Adolescent Health, 21(1)*, pp. 18–24, 1997.

Coward, R., 'Number Crunching: do Young People condone Domestic Violence?', *Guardian*, 16 February 1998.

Criminal Statistics for England and Wales. Home Office, London 1997.

Crisp, D. and Stanko, B., *Monitoring Costs and Evaluating Needs: Crime Reduction Series.* Home Office Research, Development and Statistics Directorate. London 2000.

Crisp, D. and Stanko, B., 'Monitoring Costs and Evaluating Needs', Ch. 12 in Taylor-Browne, A., *What Works in Domestic Violence? A Comprehensive Guide for Professionals.* Whiting & Birch, London 2001.

Cromwell, N. A. and Burgess, A. W., *Understanding Violence against Women.* National Academy Press, Washington DC 1996.

Crown Prosecution Service, *Policy for Prosecuting Cases of Domestic Violence.* CPS, London 1995.

Crown Prosecution Service, *Zero Tolerance for Domestic Violence.*, ref. 136/01, 28 November 2001. Available from: http://www.cps.gov.uk/

Davidson, L. L., King, V., Garcia, J. and Marchant, S., *Reducing Domestic Violence . . . What Works? Health Services.* Policing & Reducing Crime briefing note. Home Office Research, Development and Statistics Directorate. London 2000.

Davidson, L. L., King, V., Garcia, J. and Marchant, S., 'What Role can Health Services Play?'. In Taylor-Browne, J. (ed.), *What Works in Domestic Violence? A Comprehensive Guide for Professionals,* Chapter 4. Whiting & Birch, London 2001.

DeLahunta, E. A. and Tulsky, A. A., 'Personal Exposure of Faculty and Medical Students to Family Violence', *The Journal of the American Medical Association, 275(24),* pp. 1903–6, 1996.

Department of Health (DoH), 'Inspectors Report on Domestic Violence'. DoH, 96/124, London 17 April 1996.

Department of Health (DoH), *On the State of Public Health: the Annual Report of the Chief Medical Officer of the Department of Health for the Year 1996.* P23. London, HMSO 1997a.

Department of Health (DoH), *Local authority circular LAC (97)15 Family Law Act 1996. Part IV Family Homes and Domestic Violence Responsibilities of Local Authorities and the Guardian ad litem and Reporting Officer Service.* DoH, London September 1997b.

Department of Health (DoH), *Why Mothers Die. Report on Confidential Enquiries into Maternal Deaths in the United Kingdom 1994–1996.* P.159. DoH, London 1998.

Department of Health, *Working Together to Safeguard Children: a Guide to Inter-agency Working to Safeguard and Promote the Welfare of Children.* London, the Stationery Office 1999a.

Department of Health, *Responding to Families in Need: Inspection of Assessment, Management and Decision making in Family Support Services.* SSI national inspection report. DoH, London 1999b. Available from: http://www.doh.gov.uk/pdfs/familysupportreport.pdf.

Department of Health, *Domestic Violence: A Resource Manual for Health Care Professionals.* DoH, London March 2000a.

Department of Health, *Conference Report: Domestic Violence. A Health Response: Working in a Wider Partnership.* DoH, London 2000b.

Department of Health, *The Health Visitor and School Nurse Development Programme. School Nurse Practice Development Resource Pack.* DoH, London 2001.

Dobash, R. E. and Dobash, R. P., *Violence against Wives.* Free Press, New York, and Macmillan, Basingstoke 1979.

Dobash, R. E. and Dobash, R. P., *Women, Violence and Social Change.* Routledge, London 1992.

Dobash, R. E., Dobash, R. P., Cavanagh, K. and Lewis R., *Research Evaluation of Programmes for Violent Men.* The Scottish Office Central Research Unit, Edinburgh 1996.

Dobash, R. E., Dobash, R. P., Cavanagh, K. and Lewis, R., *Home Truths about Domestic Violence: Feminist Influences on Policy and Practice a Reader.* Routledge, London and New York 2000.

Domestic Abuse Intervention Project (DAIP), *Domestic Abuse Intervention Project.* 202 East Superior Street, Duluth, MN 55802, USA, 2000: http://www.duluth-model.org/daipccr3.htm

Drossman, D., Lesserman, J., Nachman, G., Zhiming, L., Gluck, H., Toomey, J. and Michell, C., 'Sexual and Physical Abuse in Women with Functional or Organic Gastrointestinal Disorders'. *Annals of Internal Medicine, 113,* pp. 828–30, 1990.

Edwards, S., *Reducing Domestic Violence . . . What Works? Use of Criminal Law*. A publication of the Policing and Reducing Crime Unit. Home Office Research, London 2000a.

Edwards, S., *Reducing Domestic Violence . . . What works? Use of Civil Law*. A publication of the Policing and Reducing Crime Unit. Home Office Research, London 2000b.

Elliott, P., 'Shattering Illusions: Same Sex Domestic Violence'. In Renzetti, C. M. and Miley, C. H. (eds,) *Violence in Gay and Lesbian Domestic Partnerships*. Sage, Newbury Park 1996.

Family Violence Prevention Fund (FVPF), *Preventing Domestic Violence: Clinical Guidelines on Routine Screening*. The Family Violence Prevention Fund's National Health Resource Center on Domestic Violence, San Francisco 1999.

Fawcett, B., Featherstone, B., Hern, J. and Toft, C. (eds), *Violence and Gender Relations: Theories and Interventions*. Sage, London 1996.

Feder, Gene, letter to *BMJ*, 2001: http://bmj.bmjjournals.com/cgi/eletters/325/7359/314 27187

Feldhaus, K. M., Koziol-McLain, J., Amsbury, H. L., Norton, I. M., Lowenstein, S. R. and Abbott, J. T., 'Accuracy of 3 Brief Screening Questions for Detecting Partner Violence in the Emergency Department', *Journal of the American Medical Association*, 277(17), pp. 1357–61, 7 May 1997.

Ferguson, C. U., 'Dating as a Social Phenomenon', Chapter 4 in Jackson and Oates' *Violence in Intimate Relationships: Examining Sociological and Psychological Issues*. Butterworth-Heinemann, Oxford and Boston 1998.

Fincham, F. D., 'Family Violence: Leonardo, Roots, Rose-coloured Glasses, and Other Observations'. In Klein, R. C. A. (ed.), *Multidisciplinary Perspectives on Family Violence*. Routledge, London and New York 2000.

Flitcraft, A., Hadley, S., Hendricks-Matthews, M. K., McLeer, S. V. and Warshaw, C., *Diagnostic Guidelines on Domestic Violence*. American Medical Association (AMA), Chicago 1992.

Frost, M., 'Clinical Issues In Domestic Violence', *Nursing Times Clinical Monograph no, 12*. E-map Healthcare Ltd. 1999.

Frost, M., 'Health Visitors' Perceptions of Domestic Violence: the Private Nature of the Problem', *Journal of Advanced Nursing, 30(3)*, pp. 589–96, September 1999.

Gaudoin, T., 'Home Truths', *The Times Magazine*, pp. 24–9, 10 November 2001.

Gerlock, A., 'Health Impact of Domestic Violence', *Issues in Mental Health Nursing*, 20, pp. 373–85, 1999.

Gibb, F., 'Legal Challenge seeks Tougher Rape Penalties' (Legal Editor), *The Times*, 13 May 2002.

Giblin, M. J., 'Catholic Church Teaching and Domestic Violence', *Journal of Religion and Culture, 34(1)*, pp. 10–21, Winter 1999.

Girshwick, L. J., 'Breaking the Silence: Sociologist Studies Woman-to-Woman Sexual Violence'. Work in progress. www.gayhealth.com

GMB, 'The Daphne Initiative (1999) a Collaborative Project to investigate the Effects of Domestic Violence in the Workplace', 2000.

Goldberg, W. and Tomlanovich, M., 'Domestic Violence Victims in the Emergency Department', *Journal of the American Medical Association*, 251, pp. 3259–64, 1984.

Gondolf, E., 'Do Batterer Programmes Work? A 15-month Follow-up of a Multi-site Evaluation', *Domestic Violence Report*, 3, June–July 1995.

Gottlieb, S., 'Doctors could have Greater Role in spotting Domestic Violence', *British Medical Journal, 317(7151)*, 11 July 1998.

Grace, S., *Policing Domestic Violence in the 1990s*. Home Office Research Study 139. Home Office, London 1995.

Graham, P., Rawlings, E. and Rimini, W., 'Survivors of the Terror: Battered Women, Hostages and the Stockholm Syndrome', in Yllo, K. and Bograd, M. (eds), *Feminist Perspectives in Wife Abuse*. Sage Publications, London 1988.

Greater London Action on Disability [GLAD]. Social Policy Research Study 81. London 1995.

Greenwich County Council, 'Domestic Violence Guidelines', Greenwich County Council, London Borough of Greenwich 2002: http://www.greenwich.gov.uk/council/ce/domv91–97.htm

Grisso, J. A., Wishner, A. R., Schwarz, D. F. and Weene, B. A., 'A Population-based Study of Injuries in Inner-city Women', *American Journal of Epidemiology, 134*, p. 59.

Hadley, S., 'Working with Battered Women in the Emergency Department: a Model Programme', *Journal of Emergency Nursing, 18*, pp. 18–23, 1992.

Hague, G., *Reducing Domestic Violence. What Works? Multi-Agency Fora.* Crime Reduction Research Series briefing note. Policing and Reducing Crime Unit, Home Office, London 2000.

Hague, G. and Malos, E., *Domestic Violence: Action for Change*, 1st edn. New Clarion Press, Cheltenham, Glos 1993.

Hague, G. and Malos, E., *Domestic Violence: Action for Change*, 2nd edn. New Clarion Press, Cheltenham, Glos 1998.

Hague, G., Mullender, A., Aris, R. and Dear, W., 'Abused Women's Perspectives: The Responsiveness of Domestic Violence Provision and Inter-Agency Initiatives', Economic and Social Research Centre (ESRC) 2001: http://www1.rhul.ac.uk/sociopolitical-science/vrp/realhome.html

Hamberger, K.L, 'Marital Violence: Batterers'. In Barnet, O. W., Miller-Perrin, C. L. and Perrin, R. D. (eds), *Family Violence Across the Lifespan: An Introduction*, Chapter 10. Sage Publications, London 1997.

Hanmer, J. and Itzin, C. (eds), *Home Truths about Domestic Violence: Feminist Influences on Policy and Practice: a Reader*. Routledge Press, London and New York 2000.

Hansard Society, 'Womenspeak: Findings of the Parliamentary Domestic Violence'. Internet Consultation, Women's Aid 2000.

Harris, J. *An evaluation of the use and effectiveness of the Protection from Harassment Act 1997*, Home Office Research Study 203; p. 13, Home Office Research Study 196. A Research, Development and Statistics Directorate Report. London: Home Office 2000.

Harris, J. and Grace, S., *A Question of Evidence? Investigating and prosecuting Rape in the 1990s*. Home Office Research Study 196. A Research, Development and Statistics Directorate report. Home Office, London 1999.

Harwin, N., Hague, G. and Malos, E., *The Multi-Agency Approach to Domestic Violence: New Opportunities, Old Challenges?* Whiting & Birch, London 1999.

Hearn, J., 'Violence towards Known Women: Men's Constructions'. In Fawcett, B., Featherstone, B., Hern, J. and Toft, C. (eds), *Violence and Gender Relations: Theories and Interventions*, Chapter 2. Sage Publications, London 1996.

Hearn, J., *The Violence of Men: How Men talk about and How Agencies respond to Men's Violence to Women*. Sage Publications, London 1996.

Heath, I., 'Domestic Violence: the General Practitioner's Role'. Royal College of General Practitioners, 2000: http://www.rcgp.org.uk/rcgp/corporate/position/dom_violence/index.asp

Henwood, M. on behalf of the Department of Health (DoH), *Domestic Violence: a Resource Manual for Health Care Professionals*. DoH, London 2000: http://www.doh.gov.uk/domestic.htm

Hester, M., Pearson, C. and Harwin, N., *Making an Impact. Children and Domestic Violence: a Reader*. Jessica Kingsley Publishers, London and Philadelphia 2000.

Hester, M. and Radford, L., 'Domestic Violence and Access Arrangements for Children in Denmark and Britain', *Journal of Social Welfare and Family Law, 1(6)*, pp. 9–12, 1992.

Hester, M. and Radford, L., 'Contradictions and Compromises: the Impact of the Children Act on Women and Children's Safety'. In Hester, M., Kelly, L. and Radford, J. (eds), *Women Violence and Male Power*. Open University Press, Milton Keynes 1996.

Holden, G. W. and Ritchie, K. L., 'Linking Extreme Marital Discord, Child Rearing and Child Behavior Problems: Evidence from Battered Women', *Child Development, 62*, pp. 311–27, 1991.

Home Office, 'Guidance to Chief Officers of Police in dealing with Domestic Violence', Circular 60/1990. Home Office, London July 1990.

Home Office, 'Interagency Co-ordination to tackle Domestic Violence'. Inter-agency circular. Home Office, London 1995.

Home Office, *Living without Fear: an Integrated Approach to tackling Violence against Women*. Home Office, London 1999.

Home Office, *Reducing Domestic Violence . . . What works?* A publication of the Policing and Reducing Crime Unit, Home Office Research. Home Office, London 2000a.

Home Office, 'Domestic Violence: Break the Chain. Multi-Agency Guidance for Addressing Domestic Violence. Home Office, London 2000b.

Home Office, 'Multi-Agency Guidance for Addressing Domestic Violence'. Home Office publications, London 2001: http://www.homeoffice.gov.uk/violenceagainstwomen

Home Office, 'Protecting the Public: Strengthening Protection against Sex Offenders and Reforming the Law on Sexual Offences', London, November 2002: http://www.protectingthepublic.homeoffice.gov.uk/PTP_Final.pdf

Hopayian, K., Horrocks, G., Garner, P. and Levitt, A., 'Battered Women presenting in General Practice', *Journal of the Royal College of General Practitioners*, 33, pp. 506–7, 1983.

Howe, A., Crilly, M. and Fairhurst, R., 'Acceptability of asking Patients about Violence in Accident and Emergency', *Emergency Medical Journal*, 19, pp. 138–40, 2002.

Huch, M. H., 'Violence against Women: a World-wide Problem', *Nursing Science Quarterly*, 340, 13(4), October 2000.

Humphreys, C., *Social Work, Domestic Violence and Child Protection: Challenging Practice*. The Policy Press, Bristol 2000a.

Humphreys, C., *Starting Over: Women and Children's Experiences of Domestic Violence Outreach*. Women's Aid Publications, Bristol 2000b.

Humphreys, C., 'Child Protection and Woman Protection: Links and Schisms. An Overview of the Research'. June 2000. WAFE web page.

Humphreys, C., Hague G., Hester, M. and Mullender, A., *Domestic Violence Good Practice Guidelines. From Good Intentions to Good Practice*. A mapping study of services working with families where there is domestic violence. Print Services, University of Warwick, Warwick 2000.

Hutchison, S. L. and Samdahl, D. M., 'Confronting Gendered Discourse in Leisure: an Added Obstacle for Women with Disabilities'. National Recreation and Parks Association Leisure Research Symposium, Miami Beach, 1 October 1998.

Ingram, R., 'Taking a Pro-active Approach: Communicating with Women Experiencing Violence from a Known Man in the Emergency Department', *Accident and Emergency Nursing*, 2, pp. 143–8, 1994.

Island D. and Lettelier, P., *Men Who Beat the Men Who Love Them*. Harrington Park Press, New York 1991.

Islington, London Borough of, *Islington Crime Survey*. London Borough of Islington, Islington 1986.

Jackson, N. A. and Oates, G. C., *Violence in Intimate Relationships: Examining Sociological and Psychological Issues*. Butterworth-Heinemann, Oxford and Boston 1998.

Jaffe, P., Wolfe, D. W. and Wilson, S. *Children of Battered Women: Issues in Child Development and Intervention Planning*. Newbury Park, CA: Sage 1990.

James-Hanman, D., 'Domestic Violence: Breaking the Chain', *Community Practitioner*, 71(12), pp. 404–7, 1998.

James-Hanman, D., 'Partnership Approaches by Agencies', Chapter 15 in Hanmer, J. and Itzin, C. (eds), *Home Truths about Domestic Violence: Feminist Influences on Policy and Practice: a Reader*. Routledge Press, London and New York 2000.

James-Hanman, D., 'Pan-London Domestic Violence Strategy', *SAFE, the domestic abuse quarterly*, Winter 2001, WAFE, Bristol. www.womensaid.co.uk

Jewish Women International, *Relationship Abuse in Jewish Homes*, 1996: http://www.jewishwomen.org/Relationship

Joseph Rowntree Foundation, *Lessons from the Domestic Violence Project (DVIP)*. JR Foundation, York 1998: http://www.jrf.org.uk.

Jukes, A., *Why Men Hate Women*. Free Association Books, London 1993.

Jukes, R., 'Editorial: Preventing Domestic Violence. Most Women Welcome Inquiries, but Doctors and Nurses Rarely Ask about it'. *British Medical Journal*, 324, pp. 253–4 (2 February) 2002; papers pp. 271, 274.

Justice for Women, *Battered Women's Syndrome: Help or Hindrance?* Justice for Women, 2002: http://www.jfw.org.uk/BWS.HT

Kashani, J., Darby, P. J., Allan, W. D., Harte, K. L. and Reid, J. C., 'Intrafamilial Homicide committed by Juveniles: Examples of a Sample with Recommendations for Prevention', *Journal of Forensic Sciences*, 42, pp. 873–8, 1997.

Kashani, J. and Wesley, A. D., 'The Impact of Family Violence on Children and Adolescents', *Developmental Clinical Psychology and Psychiatry*, 37, Sage, London 1998.

Kaufman, T., 'Domestic Violence: a Health Response', *Royal College Midwives Journal*, 3(5), 2000.

Kaufman, T., Kantor, G. and Strauss, M. A., 'The Drunken Bum Theory of Wife Beating', *Social Problems*, 34(3), pp. 186–92, 1987.

Kelly, L., *Surviving Sexual Violence*. Policy Press, Cambridge 1988.

Kelly, L., 'When Women Protection Is the Best Kind of Child Protection: Children, Domestic Violence and Child Abuse', *Administration*, 44(2), pp. 118–35, 1996.

Kelly, L., Bindel, J., Burton, S., Butterworth, D., Cook, K. and Regan, L., *Domestic Violence Matters: an Evaluation of a Development Project*. Child and Woman Abuse Studies Unit, University of North London. Home Office Research Study 193. A Research Development and Statistics Directorate Report, London 1999.

Kelly, L. and Humphreys, C., 'Supporting Women and Children in their Communities: Outreach and Advocacy Approaches to Domestic Violence'. In Taylor-Browne, J., *What Works in Domestic Violence? A Comprehensive Guide for Professionals*, Chapter 9. Whiting & Birch, London 2001.

Klein, R. C. A. (ed.), *Multidisciplinary Perspectives on Family Violence*, Routledge, London and New York 2000.

Kurz, D. and Stark, E., 'Not-so-benign Neglect: the Medical Response to Battering'. In Yllo, K. and Bograd M. (eds), *Feminist Perspectives on Wife Abuse*. Sage, London 1988.

Kyriacou, D. N., Anglin, D., Taliaferro, E., Stone S., Tubb T., Linden, J. A., Muelleman, R. B., Erik, K. and Kraus, J. F., 'Risk Factors for Injury to Women from Domestic Violence', *The New England Journal of Medicine*, 341(25), pp. 1892–8, 16 December 1999.

Lees, S., *Ruling Passions: Sexual Violence, Reputation and the Law*. Open University Press, Buckingham 1997.

Lees, S., 'Marital Rape and Marital Murder'. In Hanmer, J. and Itzin, N. (eds), *Home Truths about Domestic Violence: Feminist Influences on Policy and Practice: a Reader*. Routledge, London 2000.

Lees, S. and Gregory, J., *Rape and Sexual Assault: a Study of Attrition*. Police and Crime Prevention Unit, Islington Council, London 1993.

Letellier, P., 'Gay and Bisexual Male Domestic Violence Victimization: Challenges to Feminist Theory and Responses to Violence'. *Violence and Victims*, 9(2), pp. 95–106, 1994.

Letellier, P., 'Twin Epidemics: Domestic Violence and HIV Infection amongst Gay and Bisexual Men'. In Renzetti, C. and Miley, C. (eds), *Violence in Gay and Lesbian Domestic Partnerships* (pp. 1–19). Sage, New York 1996.

Levison, D. and Kenny, D., *The Provision of Accommodation and Support for Households Experiencing Domestic Violence in England*. London Research Centre. Office of the Deputy Prime Minister, London December 2002.

Lockton, D. and Ward, R., *Domestic Violence*. Cavendish Publishing, London 1997.

Mama, A., *The Hidden Struggle: Statutory and Voluntary Sector Responses to Violence against Black Women in the Home*. Whiting & Birch, London 1996.

Mama, A., 'Black Women in the Home'. In Hanmer, J. and Itzin, C. (eds), *Home Truths about Domestic Violence: Feminist Influences on Policy and Practice, a Reader*, Chapter 3. Routledge Press, London 2000.

Marchant, S., Davidson, L. L., Garcia, J. and Parsons, J. E., 'Addressing Domestic Violence through Maternity Services: Policy and Practice', *Midwifery*, *17(3)*, September 2001.

Mayhew, P., Mirlees-Black, C. and Percy, A., *The 1996 British Crime Survey England & Wales*. Home Office Statistical Bulleting, Issue 19.96. Home Office, London 1996.

McGee, C., *Children's Experience of Domestic Violence*. National Society for the Prevention of Cruelty to Children, London 1996.

McGee, C., 'Children's Experiences of Domestic Violence', *Child and Family Social Work*, 2, pp. 32–5, 1997.

McGee, C., 'Children's and Mothers' Experiences of Support and Protection following Domestic Violence', In Hanmer, J. and Itzin, C. (eds), *Home Truths about Domestic Violence: Feminist Influences on Policy and Practice: a Reader*, Chapter 5. Routledge, London and New York 2000a.

McGee, C., *Childhood Experiences of Domestic Violence*. Jessica Kingsley Publisher, London 2000b.

McGibbon, A. and Kelly, L., *Abuse of Women in the Home: Advice and Information*. London Borough of Hammersmith and Fulham. London 1989.

McPherson, H. C., 'Domestic Violence: Planning Your Way to Safety', *View*, *36(6)*, pp. 24–7, 1994.

Memon, K., 'Wife Abuse in the Muslim Community', Belfast Islamic Centre: http://www.khyber.demon.co.uk/comfort/articles/abuse/htm

Metropolitan Police Service (MPS), *'Enough is Enough'*. MPS Domestic Violence Strategy, London 2001: www.met.police.uk/enoughisenough/strategy.htm

Metropolitan Police Service (MPS), 'High Risk Factors for Domestic Violence Murders Identified'. Bulletin 2002/0248 23, December 2002: http://www.met.police.uk/pns/DisplayPN.cqi?pn id=2002 0248.

Meyer, H., 'The Billion Dollar Epidemic', *American Medical News*, 6 January 1992.

Mezey, G., 'Domestic Violence in Health Settings', *Current Opinion in Psychiatry*, *14(6)*, pp. 543–7, Lippincott, Williams & Wilkins, London November 2001.

Mezey, G. and Bewley, G.C., 'Domestic Violence and Pregnancy: Risk Is Greatest after Delivery' [Editorial], *British Medical Journal*, *314(7090)*, p. 1295, 3 May 1997.

Mezey, G., Bacchus, L., Bewley, S. and Haworth, A., *An Exploration of the Prevalence, Nature and Effects of Domestic Violence in Pregnancy*. ESRC, Violence Research Programme, Holloway, London 2001.

Mignon, S.I., 'Husband Battering: a Review of the Debate over a Controversial Social Phenomenon. In Jackson, A. J. and Oates, G. C., *Violence in Intimate Relationships: Examining Sociological and Psychological Issues*, Chapter 6. Butterworth-Heinemann, Oxford and Boston 1998.

Miller, B. A., Wilsnack, S. C. and Cunradi, C. B., 'Family Violence and Victimization: Treatment Issues for Women with Alcohol Problems', *Alcoholism: Clinical and Experimental Research*, *24(8)*, pp. 1287–1297, Lippincott Williams & Wilkins, London and New York August 2000.

Mirrlees-Black, M. C., *Domestic Violence: Findings from a new British Crime Survey Self-completion Questionnaire*. Home Office Research Study 191. Research, Development and Statistics Directorate, London 1999.

Mirrlees-Black, M. C. and Byron, M., *Domestic Violence: Findings from the BCS Self-Completion Questionnaire*. Home Office Research Study no 86. Research, Development and Statistics Directorate, London 1999.

Mooney, J., *The Hidden Figure: Domestic Violence in North London*. Police and Crime Prevention Unit, Islington Council 1993. Middlesex University Centre for Criminology, London 1994.

Mooney, J., 'Revealing the Hidden Figure of Domestic Violence'. In Hanmer, J. and Itzin, C. (eds), *Home Truths about Domestic Violence: Feminist Influences on Policy and Practice, a Reader*, Routledge, London and New York 2000.

Moore, M. L., 'Attitudes and Practices of Registered Nurses toward Women Who Have Experienced Abuse/Domestic Violence', *Journal of Obstetric, Gynaecologic, & Neonatal Nursing, 27(2)*, pp. 175–82, March/April 1998.

Morgan, J., *Conference News from the Royal College of Midwives*. Bournemouth Bulletin. Wednesday 1 May 2002.

Morley, R. and Mullender, A., *Preventing Domestic Violence to Women*. Police Research Group Crime Prevention Unit Series: Paper No. 48. Home Office Police Department, London 1994.

Mullender, A., *Rethinking Domestic Violence: The Social Work and Probation Response*. Routledge, London 1996.

Mullender, A., *Reducing Domestic Violence . . . What Works? Meeting the Needs of Children*. Crime Reduction Series. Policing and Reducing Crime Unit, Home Office, London January 2000.

Mullender, A. and Burton, S., *Reducing Domestic Violence . . . What Works? Perpetrator Programmes*. Crime Reduction Series, Policing and Reducing Crime Unit, Home Office, London January 2000.

Mullender, A., Kelly, L., Hague, G., Malos, E. and Imam, U., *Children's Needs, Coping Strategies and Understanding of Woman Abuse*. Full report of research activities and results. award No. L129 25 1037, 2001.

Myhill, A. and Allen, J., *Rape and Sexual Assault of Women: the Extent and Nature of the Problem*. Findings from the British Crime Survey. Home Office Research Study 237. Home Office Research, Development and Statistics Directorate, London, March 2002.

Naffine, N., 'Possession: Erotic Love in the Law of Rape'. *Modern Law Review, 57(1)*, Blackwell, London January 1994.

National Association for Domestic Violence Perpetrator Programmes and Associated Support, 'Statement of Principles of the National Practitioners Association, 2000. RESPECT, c/o DVIP, PO Box 2838, London W6 9ZE: http://www.domesticviolencedata.org/7-resources_pdf/respect.pdf

National Center for Injury Prevention and Control, *Dating Violence*. NCIPC, Atlanta, CA January 2000.

National Clearinghouse for Alcohol and Drug Information, US Department of Health and Human Services, Public Health Service, Substance Abuse and Mental Health Services Administration, Center for Substance Abuse Treatment, 102 pp., 1997: http://www.health.org/catalog/catalog.htm

Newberger, E. H., Barkan, S. E., McCormick, M. C., Yllo, K., Gary, L. T. and Schecter, S., 'Abuse of Pregnant Women and Adverse Birth Outcome: Current Knowledge and Implications for Practices', *Journal of the American Medical Association, 267*, pp. 2370–2, 1992.

North Thames Region, 'National Guidelines on the Management of Adult Victims of Sexual Assault: an Adaptation of the UK National Guidelines on Sexually Transmitted Infections and Closely Related Conditions, 1998.

Nosek, M. A, Howland, C. A. and Young, M. E., 'Abuse of Women with Disabilities: Policy Implications', *Journal of Disability Policy Studies*, 8, pp. 157–76, 1997.

Nosek, M., *Dispelling the Myth: 'No one would ever abuse a woman with a disability'*. Center for Research on Women with Disabilities. Houston, TX 1999: http://www.bcm.tmc.edu/crowd/index.htm

Nursing and Midwifery Council, Code of Professional Conduct for Nurses, Midwives and Health Visitors, 2002: www.nmc-uk.org

Oates, G. C., 'Cultural Perspectives on Intimate Violence'. In Jackson, N. A. and Oates, G. C., *Violence in Intimate Relationships: Examining Sociological and Psychological Issues*, Chapter 10. Butterworth-Heinemann, Oxford and Boston MA 1998.

O'Dowd, T. and Jewell, D., *Men's Health*. Oxford University Press, Oxford/London 1998.

Office of the Deputy Prime Minister, *Supporting People: Handy Guide*. Addressing domestic violence in the 'Supporting People' programme. London December 2002: www.odpm.gov.uk

O'Rourke, M., Hammond, S. and Bucknall, M., *Multi-Agency Risk Management: Safeguarding Public Safety and Individual Care*. Risk Assessment, Management and Audit systems. DoH, London January 2001.

Pahl, J., 'Health Professionals and Violence Against Women'. In Kingston, P. and Penhale, B (eds), *Family Violence and the Caring Professions*. Macmillan, London 1995.

Painter, K., *Wife Rape, Marriage and the Law. Survey Report: Key Findings and Recommendations*. Department of Social Policy and Social Work, University of Manchester, Manchester 1991.

Parsons, L. H., Zaccaro, D., Wells, B., Stovall, T. G., Pearse, W. H. and Horger, E. O., 'Methods of and Attitudes toward Screening Obstetrics and Gynaecology Patients for Domestic Violence'. *American Journal of Obstetrics and Gynaecology, 173(2)*, pp. 381–7, 1995.

Peckover, S., 'Domestic Violence: On the Health Visiting Agenda?', *Community Practitioner, 71(12)*, pp. 408–9, 1998.

Peckover, S., 'Domestic Abuse and Women's Health: the Challenge for Primary Care', *Primary Health Care Research and Development, 3(3)*, pp. 151–8(8), 1 July 2002.

Peckover, S., Marshall, K. and Kendall, S., *Understanding Domestic Violence: a Training Pack for Community Practitioners*. Community Practitioners' and Health Visitors Association, London 2001: www.msfcphva.org.

Ptacek, J., 'Why Do Men Batter Their Wives'. In Yllö, K. and Bograd, M., *Feminist Perspective on Wife Abuse*. Sage, Newbury Park, CA 1988

Public and Commercial Services Union [PCSU]: http://www.pcs.org.uk/equality/briefings/domviolguide.htm

Radford, L. and Cappel, C., *Domestic Violence and the Methodist Church – the Way Forward*. Conference Report. Methodist Women's Network and the Church's Family and Personal Relationships Committee, Methodist Church 2001.

Ramsay, J., Richardson, J., Carter, Y., Davidson, L. L. and Feder, G., 'Should Health Professionals Screen Women for Domestic Violence? Systematic Review', *British Medical Journal, 325(7359)*, p. 314, 10 August 2002.

Rape Crisis Federation for England & Wales, 'Police Reporting, Court Procedures and the Law', 2001: http://www.rapecrisis.co.uk/policereporting.htm

Rapkin, A., Kames, L., Darke, L., Stampler, F. and Naliboff, B., 'History of Physical and Sexual Abuse in Women with Chronic Pelvic Pain', *Obstetrics and Gynecology, 76*, pp. 92–5, 1990.

Ratner, P., 'Indicators of Exposure to Wife Abuse', *Canadian Journal of Nursing Research, 27(1)*, pp. 31–46, 1995.

Renzetti, C. M., Edleson, J. L. and Kennedy-Bergen, R., *Sourcebook on Violence against Women*. Sage, London 2001.

Rhee, S., 'Domestic Violence in the Korean Immigrant Family', *Journal of Sociology & Social Welfare, 24(1)*, pp. 163–77, 1997.

Richardson, J., Coid, C., Petruckevitch, A., Chung, W. A., Moorey, A. and Feder, G., 'Identifying Domestic Violence: Cross-sectional Study in Primary Care', *British Medical Journal, 324, 274*, 2 February 2002.

Roberts, A. R., *Crisis Intervention Handbook: Assessment, Treatment and Research*, 2nd edn. Oxford University Press, Oxford/London 2000.

Roche, B., *Domestic Violence: Raising Awareness*. The Cabinet Office, Domestic Violence Home Page, London 2002: http://www.cabinet-office.gov.uk/index.htm

Römkens, R. and Mastenbroek, S., 'Budding Happiness. The Relationship Dynamics of the Abuse of Girls and Young Women by their Boyfriends'. In Klein, C. A., *Multidisciplinary Perspectives in Family Violence*, Chapter 4. Routledge, London 1998.

Royal College of Midwives, 'Domestic Abuse In Pregnancy', Position Paper No 19a. Royal College of Midwives, London March 1999: http://www.rcm.org.uk

Royal College of Nursing, *Domestic Violence: Guidance for Nurses*. LRC, London 2000.

Royal College of Obstetricians and Gynaecologists, 'Confidentiality and Disclosure of Health Information', RCOG Ethics Committee comments on a BMA document, 1997. Available from Royal College of Obstetricians and Gynaecologists, 27 Sussex Place, Regent's Park, London NW1 4RG.

Royal College of Psychiatrists, 'Rape', Council Report CR47. London, March 1996.

Rusell, P., Dobash, R., Dobash, E., Cavanagh, K. and Lewis, R., 'Confronting Violent Men'. In Hanmer, J. and Itzin, C. (eds), *Home Truths about Domestic Violence: Feminist Influences on Policy and Practice, a Reader*. Routledge Press, London and New York 2000.

Salber, P. R. and Taliaferro, E., *The Physician's Guide to Domestic Violence*. Volcano Press, Volcano, CA, 1995.

Santa Clara County, 'Santa Clara County Domestic Violence Protocol for Health Providers'. Santa Clara County Domestic Violence Council, Santa Clara County Board of Supervisors, Santa Clara Valley Medical Center 1997.

Shepherd, J. P., 'Violent Crime: an Accident and Emergency Perspective', *British Journal of Criminology*, 30, pp. 280–305, 1990.

Shepherd, J. P., 'Tackling Violence – an Editorial', *British Medical Journal*, 316, pp. 879–80 21 March 1998.

Shepherd, J. P., *Violence in Health Care: Understanding and Surviving Violence: a Practical Guide for Health Professionals*. Oxford University Press, Oxford/London 2001.

Shipway, L., *Facilitating Survivors of Domestic Violence and Sexual Assault – an Open Learning Package*. Anglia Polytechnic University, Chelmsford 1996.

Shornstein, S., *Domestic Violence and Health Care: 'What Every Health Professional Needs to Know'*. Sage, London 1997.

Sipe, B. and Hall, E.J., *'I Am Not Your Victim'*: Anatomy of Domestic Violence. Sage, London 1996.

Smith, F., in consultation with Lyon, Professor T., *Domestic Violence (Part IV Family Law Act 1996 & Protection from Harassment Act 1997)* Children Act Enterprises, London 1998.

Smith, L., *Domestic Violence: An Overview of the Literature*. Home Office Research Study No. 107. Her Majesty's Stationery Office, London 1989.

Stanko, E. A. (ed.), *Taking Stock: What Do We Know bout Violence?* ESCR Violence Research Project. HMSO, London 1998.

Stanko, E., Crisp, D., Hale, C. and Lucraft, H., *Counting the Cost: Estimating the Impact of Domestic Violence in the London Borough of Hackney*. Crime Concern, London 1997.

Stark, E. and Flitcraft, A., *Women at Risk: Domestic Violence and Women's Health*. Sage, London 1996.

Stark, E., Flitcraft, A. and Frazier, W., 'Medicine and Patriarchal Violence: the Social Construction of a "Private Event"', *Int. Journal of Health Services*, 9(3), pp. 461–93, 1979.

Stelman, A. E., Johnson, B., Hanley, S. and Geraghty, J., 'The Probation Perspective'. In Harwin, N., Hague, G. and Malos, E., *The Multi-Agency Approach to Domestic Violence: New Opportunities, Old Challenges?*, Chapter 15. Whiting & Birch, London 1999.

Stevens, K. L. H., 'The Role of the Accident and Emergency Department', in Bewley, S., Friend, J. and Mezey, G. (eds), *Violence against Women*. London, Royal College of Obstetricians and Gynaecologists, 1997.

Straus, M.A., 'Measuring Intra-family Conflict and Violence: the Conflict Tactics Scale (CTS)', *Journal of Marriage and the Family*, 41, pp. 75–88, 1979.

Sugg, N.K. and Inui, T., 'Primary Care Physicians' Response to Domestic Violence: Opening Pandora's Box', *JAMA*, 7, pp. 3157–60, 1992.

Summers, R. W. and Hoffman, A. M., *Domestic Violence: a Global View*. Greenwood Press, London 2002.

Tarling, R., Dowds, L. and Budd, T., *Victim and Witness Intimidation: Key Findings from the British Crime Survey*. Home Office RDSD Research Findings No. 124. London 2000.

Taylor-Browne, J. (ed.), *What Works in Domestic Violence? A Comprehensive Guide for Professionals.* Whiting & Birch, London 2001.

Tilden, V. P., Schmidt, T. A., Limandri, B. J., Chiodo G. T., Garland, M. J. and Loveless, P. A., 'Factors that Influence a Clinician's Assessment and Management of Family Violence', *American Journal of Public Health, 84(4)*, pp. 628–33, 1994.

Trades Union Congress, 'Breaking the Silence on Domestic Violence', a report on the delegate surveys and workshops at the TUC Women's Conference 2002, issued 27 June 2002: http://www.tuc.org.uk/equality/tuc-5112-f0.cfm

Victim Support, *Domestic Violence: Report of a National Inter-Agency Working Party on Domestic Violence* [convened by Victim Support]. Victim Support, London 1992.

Victim Support, 2002: http://www.victimsupport-mk.org.uk/publications.htm

WAFE, *see* Women's Aid Federation of England.

Walby, S. and Mayhill, A., *Assessing and Managing the Risk of Domestic Violence: a Briefing Note.* Crime Reduction Research Series. Policing and Reducing Crime Unit, Home Office, London 2000.

Walker, L., *The Battered Woman Syndrome.* Springer Press, New York 1984.

Walklate, S., *Victimology.* Unwin Hyman, London 1989.

Wallace, H. *Family Violence: Legal, Medical, and Social Perspectives.* New York: Simon & Schuster, 280–283, 1996.

Warsaw, C. and Alpert, E., 'Integrating Routine Inquiry about Domestic Violence into Daily Practice' [Editorial], *Annals of Internal Medicine, 131(8)*, pp. 619–20, 19 October 1999.

Warshaw, C., 'Limitations of the Medical Model in the Care of Battered Women'. In Bart, P. and Moran, E. (eds), *Violence against Women: the Bloody Footprints.* Sage, London 1993.

Watson, J. and Healy, C., *Domestic Violence: Guidelines for Health Professionals*, (Pilot Draft). Camden & Islington Health Authority and Camden Multi-Agency Domestic Violence Forum, London August 1998.

Webb, E., Shankleman, J., Evans, M. R. and Brooks, R., 'The Health of Children in Refuges for Women Victims of Domestic Violence: Cross-sectional Descriptive Survey', *British Medical Journal, 323*, 28 July 2001.

Whately, M.A., 'For Better for Worse: the Case of Marital Rape', *Violence and Victims*, 8, pp. 29–39, 1993.

Wiehe, V.R., *Understanding Family Violence: Treating and Preventing Partner, Child, Sibling and Elder Abuse.* Sage, London 1998.

Williamson, E., *Domestic Violence & Health: The Response of the Medical Profession.* Policy Press, London 2000.

Wilson, E., *What's to Be Done about Domestic Violence against Women?* Penguin, London 1983.

Women's Aid Federation of England, 'The Effects of Domestic Violence on Children', Domestic Violence statistical factsheet – Children, August 1999.

Women's Aid Federation of England, 'WAFE Web Resources Page', Women's Aid Federation of England 2001: www.womensaid.co.uk

Women's Aid Federation of England, *The Domestic Abuse Quarterly*, WAFE, Bristol, Winter 2001: www.womensaid.co.uk

Women's Aid Federation of England, Briefing: Response to the 2002 Criminal Justice White Paper 'Justice for All', 2003: www.womensaid.org.uk

Women's Aid Federation of England, 2002: http://www.womensaid.org.uk/search/contents.htm

Wood, G. G. and Middleman, R., 'Re-casting the Die: a Small Group Approach to Giving Batterers a Chance to Change'. Paper presented at the 10th Annual Symposium on Social Work with Groups, Miami, FA, October 1990.

World Medical Association, 'Declaration on Family Violence', adopted by the 48th General Assembly, South Africa, October 1996.

Yick, A. G. and Agbayani-Siewert, P., 'Perception of Domestic Violence in a Chinese American Community', *Journal of Interpersonal Violence*, *12(6)*, pp. 832–46, 1997.

Yoshioka, M. R. and Dang, Q., 'Asian Task Force Against Domestic Violence, Inc.', Boston, MA, 2000: available from: www.atask.org

Young, H., Stafford, J. and Chadwick, R., *Working together to Reduce Crime. Tackling Domestic Violence*. Crime Concern. Home Office, London 2001: http://www.crimeconcern.org.uk or visit: http://www.crimereduction.gov.uk

Young, M. E.,Nosek, M. A., Howland, C. A., Chanpong, G. and Rintala, D. H., 'Prevalence of Abuse of Women with Physical Disabilities', *Archives of Physical Medicine and Rehabilitation*, *78* (Suppl.), S34–S38, 1997.

Index